AF830651

Iran's Foreign Policy

This book analyzes both domestic and international factors that have influenced *Iran's foreign policy* since 1979. It looks not only at the perspectives of the ruling elite, but also of civil society and opposition groups. Furthermore, it also analyzes the interactions among Iran's policies and those of regional and global powers.

Since the 1979 revolution, *Iran's foreign policy* has appeared both threatening and puzzling. Some have described it as ideological, whereby the regime has been attempting to export its Islamist rule to neighboring countries and challenging the international order. Others consider *Iran's foreign policy* to be primarily pragmatic, concerned with survival of the regime and expanding its power not unlike other powers in the system. This book attempts to go deeper than most conventional analyses. It demystifies *Iran's foreign policy* by describing, in great detail, foreign policy decision making in Iran. Iran is not a one-man dictatorship. Rather, it is rule by an oligarchy of Shia fundamentalists. The regime's ideology has not been cohesive, nor has it remained consistent in the past 41 years, nor all members of the ruling oligarchy have articulated an identical version of it. The book describes foreign policies of various factions and their leading figures as well as analyzing their evolutions since 1979. It explains how various intra-elite configurations of power have influenced the regime's foreign policy regarding the nuclear weapons program and the relations with the U.S.

Iran's Foreign Policy: Elite Factionalism, Ideology, the Nuclear Weapons Program, and the United States adds fresh and critical perspectives on scholarly and policy debates on *Iran's foreign policy.*

The chapters in this book were originally published in the following journals: *Comparative Strategy*, *American Foreign Policy Interests*, and the *Terrorism Law Report*.

Masoud Kazemzadeh is Associate Professor, Department of Political Science, Sam Houston State University, Huntsville, USA. He received his BA in international relations from the University of Minnesota, USA, and his MA and PhD in political science from the University of Southern California, Los Angeles, USA. He was a postdoctoral fellow at Harvard University's Center for Middle Eastern Studies.

Iran's Foreign Policy

Elite Factionalism, Ideology, the Nuclear Weapons Program, and the United States

Masoud Kazemzadeh

Routledge
Taylor & Francis Group
LONDON AND NEW YORK

First published 2020
by Routledge
2 Park Square, Milton Park, Abingdon, Oxon, OX14 4RN

and by Routledge
52 Vanderbilt Avenue, New York, NY 10017

Routledge is an imprint of the Taylor & Francis Group, an informa business

© 2020 Taylor & Francis

Chapter 3 © 2020 National Committee on American Foreign Policy
Chapter 4 © 2020 National Committee on American Foreign Policy

All rights reserved. No part of this book may be reprinted or reproduced or utilised in any form or by any electronic, mechanical, or other means, now known or hereafter invented, including photocopying and recording, or in any information storage or retrieval system, without permission in writing from the publishers.

Trademark notice: Product or corporate names may be trademarks or registered trademarks, and are used only for identification and explanation without intent to infringe.

British Library Cataloguing-in-Publication Data
A catalogue record for this book is available from the British Library

ISBN13: 978-0-367-49545-9

Typeset in Minion Pro
by codeMantra

Publisher's Note
The publisher accepts responsibility for any inconsistencies that may have arisen during the conversion of this book from journal articles to book chapters, namely the inclusion of journal terminology.

Disclaimer
Every effort has been made to contact copyright holders for their permission to reprint material in this book. The publishers would be grateful to hear from any copyright holder who is not here acknowledged and will undertake to rectify any errors or omissions in future editions of this book.

For Penny, my partner in crime, with love.

Contents

	Citation Information	viii
	Acknowledgments	ix
	Introduction	1
1	Foreign policy decision making in Iran and the nuclear program	3
2	Ayatollah Khamenei's Foreign Policy Orientation	20
3	Hassan Rouhani's Election and Its Consequences for American Foreign Policy	36
4	The Perils and Costs of a Grand Bargain with the Islamic Republic of Iran	47
5	The sources of the Middle East's crises and American grand strategy	74
6	U.S.–Iran Confrontation in the Post-NIE World: An Analysis of Alternative Policy Options	90
7	U.S.–Iran Confrontation: Domestic Asymmetrical Ramifications	113
	Index	117

Citation Information

The chapters in this book were originally published in *Comparative Strategy* and *American Foreign Policy Interests*. When citing this material, please use the original page numbering for each article, as follows:

Chapter 1
Foreign policy decision making in Iran and the nuclear program
Masoud Kazemzadeh
Comparative Strategy, volume 36, issue 3 (2017) pp. 198–214

Chapter 2
Ayatollah Khamenei's Foreign Policy Orientation
Masoud Kazemzadeh
Comparative Strategy, volume 32, issue 5 (2013) pp. 443–458

Chapter 3
Hassan Rouhani's Election and Its Consequences for American Foreign Policy
Masoud Kazemzadeh
American Foreign Policy Interests, volume 36, issue 2 (2014) pp. 127–137

Chapter 4
The Perils and Costs of a Grand Bargain with the Islamic Republic of Iran
Masoud Kazemzadeh
American Foreign Policy Interests, volume 29, issue 5 (2007) pp. 301–327

Chapter 5
The sources of the Middle East's crises and American grand strategy
Masoud Kazemzadeh
Comparative Strategy, volume 37, issue 1 (2018) pp. 56–72

Chapter 6
U.S.–Iran Confrontation in the Post-NIE World: An Analysis of Alternative Policy Options
Masoud Kazemzadeh
Comparative Strategy, volume 28, issue 1 (2009) pp. 37–59

For any permission-related enquiries please visit:
http://www.tandfonline.com/page/help/permissions

Acknowledgments

This book is the fruit of a research project that began in 2004, when I was at Utah Valley University. I thank my former department chair and friend, Dr. Keith Snedegar, who provided class releases so that I could conduct the basic research. I also thank my former Dean and friend, Dr. William Cobb, for the generous Dean's Scholarship so that I could afford to do so.

I have published the results of my research in a number of scholarly journals. All the chapters in this book have been previously published at *Comparative Strategy*, *American Foreign Policy Interests*, and *Terrorism Law Report*.

I thank Dr. Steve Lambakis for kindly granting permission to republish four of my articles. They are as follows:

Chapter 1: "Foreign Policy Decision Making in Iran and the Nuclear Program." *Comparative Strategy* (2017), 36 (3): 198–214.

Chapter 2: "Ayatollah Khamenei's Foreign Policy Orientation." *Comparative Strategy* (2013), 32 (5): 443–458.

Chapter 5: "The Sources of the Middle East's Crises and American Grand Strategy." *Comparative Strategy* (2018), 37 (1): 56–72.

Chapter 6: "U.S.-Iran Confrontation in the Post-NIE World: An Analysis of Alternative Policy Options." *Comparative Strategy* (2009), 28 (1): 37–59.

I thank Dr. George Schwab, Ambassador Susan Elliott, and Stephen Whittaker at the National Committee on American Foreign Policy and the *American Foreign Policy Interests* for kindly granting me permission to republish the following:

Chapter 3: "Hassan Rouhani's Election and its Consequences for American Foreign Policy." *American Foreign Policy Interests* (2014), 36 (2): 127–137.

Chapter 4: "The Perils and Costs of a Grand Bargain with the Islamic Republic of Iran." *American Foreign Policy Interests* (2007), 29 (5): 301–327.

The final chapter was published at *Terrorism Law Report* (now defunct), which was published by the Center for Terrorism Law at St. Mary's University School of Law, San Antonio, USA.

Chapter 7: "U.S.-Iran Confrontation: Domestic Asymmetrical Ramifications." *Terrorism Law Report* (2012), 4 (1).

This book is based on theories of Foreign Policy Analysis (FPA). I owe great debts to two top scholars of FPA theories: Valerie M. Hudson and James N. Rosenau. I thank Dr. Hudson for reading many of the chapters in this book and providing her suggestions and criticisms. She was amazingly kind and generous with her time and suggestions. I have also benefitted enormously from the late Dr. Rosenau's insights. I was his student at the University of Southern California. I am solely responsible for any errors of fact or interpretation.

Introduction

Since the 1979 revolution, Iran's foreign policy has appeared both threatening and puzzling. Some have described it as ideological, whereby the regime has been attempting to export its Islamist rule to neighboring countries and challenging the international order. Others consider Iran's foreign policy to be primarily pragmatic, concerned with survival of the regime and expanding its power not unlike other powers in the system. This book attempts to go deeper than most conventional analyses.

In this book, I attempt to explain and demystify Iran's foreign policy by describing, in great detail, its foreign policy decision making. Iran is not a one-man dictatorship. Rather, it is ruled by an oligarchy comprised of fundamentalist Shia clerics and lay fundamentalists.

In Chapter 1, I demonstrate how foreign policy is formulated and conducted by analyzing the roles of factions and their leaders within various institutions and offices such as the Supreme Leader, Presidency, Supreme National Security Council, and the Islamic Revolutionary Guards Corps (IRGC). The role and power of each of these offices has ebbed and flowed since 1979. I situate the evolution of these offices within the struggles among various factions and their leaders.

I show that the regime's ideology has not been cohesive, nor has it remained consistent since 1979, nor all members of the ruling oligarchy have articulated an identical version of it. The chapter describes views and foreign policy proposals of various factions and their leading figures as well as analyzes their evolutions since 1979. It analyzes how various intra-elite configurations of power have influenced the regime's foreign policy regarding the nuclear weapons program, relations with the U.S., and Iran's regional policies. Although the 1979 Constitution and the 1989 revised Constitution gave the office of the Supreme Leader enormous powers, Ayatollah Ali Khamenei, who ascended to that office in 1989, has had to struggle with other members of the oligarchy for exercising actual power to make binding decisions. He has not always been successful. At many junctures, he has had to acquiesce to the wishes of other members of the oligarchy.

In Chapter 2, I analyze the foreign policy orientation of the most powerful figure in the Islamic Republic of Iran (IRI): Supreme Leader Ayatollah Ali Khamenei. I show that both ends and means in the regime's foreign policy contain both ideological and pragmatic elements. In other words, perspectives that argue that the Islamic Republic's foreign policy is either ideological or pragmatic are over-simplifications. This chapter demonstrates the ideological (Shia fundamentalist) and pragmatic elements in both the ends and means of IRI's foreign policy. Moreover, I show that some of the elements are consistent with Shia fundamentalists ideology but not with a secular rationality.

Chapter 3 attempts to provide a more nuanced analysis of the foreign policy of a major faction within the fundamentalist oligarchy through analyzing the views and policies of Hojatolislam Hassan Rouhani, one of the leading figures in the regime since 1979. Much of the scholarly, policy, and journalistic works on Iran tend to either exaggerate the differences among the fundamentalist elites or totally dismiss them. This chapter builds upon the materials presented in Chapters 1 and 2, and shows both similarities and differences among the elites ruling Iran.

This book analyzes both domestic and international factors that have influenced Iran's foreign policy since 1979. It looks not only at the perspectives of the ruling elite, but also the perspectives of civil society and opposition groups. In Chapter 4, I analyze the interactions among Iran's policies and those of regional and global powers as well as the views of Iran's main opposition groups.

Chapter 5 further expands the analysis of Iran's foreign policy by situating it within broader grand historical transformations that have been occurring in the Middle East and North Africa in the past 100 plus years. The fundamentalist regime is both a product of these transformations and a major spur to some of them. This chapter argues that there are four major crises convulsing the Middle East. They are the Shia-Sunni conflict, rise of extremist militant fundamentalists (both Shia and Sunni), ethno-national demands, and pro-democracy movements. These have given rise to four clusters of actors. The chapter analyzes the ideological sources of Sunni and Shia fundamentalism as well as Iran's grand strategy and American strategies and policies since 1979 trying to respond to these crises and challenges. It discusses the reasons for successes and failures of American policies and identifies lessons for future American policies toward the Middle East.

In Chapter 6, I present diverse policy options as well as discuss and analyze their consequences for various actors. This chapter does not recommend one particular policy. It does, however, analyze which options and policies would be the worst-case scenarios for some or all players.

In Chapter 7, I argue that a potential war between the U.S. and Iran would, in all likelihood, contain major asymmetrical elements. In its conflicts with others, the fundamentalist regime has utilized terrorism and hostage-taking as tools of statecraft. Utilizing its previous clandestine actions, I show what might be some likely actions that the fundamentalist regime may carry out inside the U.S.

In this book, I use the term "fundamentalist regime" for "*Nizam Velayat Faqih.*" The literal translation would be the "system of rule by a high-ranking Shia cleric." This system was established by Ayatollah Ruhollah Khomeini in Iran after the 1979 revolution.

I use the term "fundamentalists" for the supporters of Khomeini and his regime. This includes the officials and supporters of the Islamic Republican Party (IRP). Between February 1979 and June 1981, many non-fundamentalists were part of the post-revolution governing structure. For example, liberal Islamist Liberation Movement of Iran, under the leadership of Mehdi Bazargan, who served as the Prime Minister in the provisional government, was a main element within the governing structure. Also the first elected President was Dr. Abol-Hassan Bani-Sadr, a progressive liberal Islamist. The non-fundamentalists also included the secular liberal democrats and secular social democrats of the Iran National Front under the leadership of Dr. Karim Sanjabi. All the non-fundamentalists were purged from positions of power by June 1981. The fundamentalists then eliminated many non-fundamentalist groups and individuals (e.g., Marxists, left-wing Islamists, and ethnic minority parties) through violence and mass executions.

I use the term "fundamentalist oligarchy" to refer to those who supported Khomeini's interpretation of Islam and were officials in the post-June 1981 regime. The IRP soon split into three main factions: left, center, and right. Around 1997, the left faction of the fundamentalist oligarchy (e.g., Mohammad Khatami, Mir Hussein Mousavi, and Mehdi Karroubi) chose the name "reformist," while the right faction (e.g., Ali Khamenei) became known as "hard-liners" or "principlists." The center faction (e.g., Ali Akbar Rafsanjani and Hassan Rouhani) became known as "moderates," or "pragmatic conservatives," or "expedients." Some fundamentalists use the term "*khodi*" [of one's own] to refer to the members of the fundamentalist oligarchy and use the term "*gher-e khodi*" [not of one's own] to refer to non-fundamentalists.

The first three chapters present domestic and foreign policies of each faction and its leaders as well as their evolutions since 1979. All the chapters attempt to explain the complex interactions of domestic and international factors in the making of Iran's foreign policy. This book hopes to add fresh perspectives on scholarly and policy debates on Iran's foreign policy.

Foreign policy decision making in Iran and the nuclear program

Masoud Kazemzadeh

ABSTRACT
This article analyzes how foreign policy is made in the Islamic Republic of Iran. To do so, it analyzes the role of various state institutions, factions, and individuals in the formulation and conduct of foreign policy. Actual powers of various institutions in Iran have evolved greatly since 1979. The history and causes of such institutional changes are discussed briefly. Iran is not a one-man dictatorship. Rather, it is ruled by an oligarchy comprised of fundamentalist Shia clerics and lay fundamentalists. The ruling elite is composed of competing factions such as hard-liners, expedients, and reformists, as well as sub-factions such as pragmatic hard-liners and ultra-hard-liners. The oligarchy is deeply divided on many issues, including on foreign policy. This article presents, in great detail, the views and policy proposals of the top members of the oligarchy regarding Iran's nuclear program, relations with the U.S., and Iran's regional policies. Finally, this article applies the findings of this research to the case of Iran's nuclear program. Evidence shows that Iran has had a clandestine nuclear weapons program. This article analyzes the ruling oligarchy's responses to the global reaction to Iran's nuclear program.

How is foreign policy made in the Islamic Republic of Iran? The political system in Iran is complex, opaque, and mystifying. Many observers are perplexed by the divergent, even contradictory, voices coming from Tehran on vital foreign policy issues. To many it is not clear who makes foreign policy in Iran.

Theories of foreign policy analysis

The subfield of foreign policy analysis (FPA) provides theories, cues, and guidelines for answering how foreign policy is made in Iran. Generally speaking, the agent-specific theories of FPA are useful in outlining an approach to the study of Iranian foreign policy decision making.[1] Human beings, and not abstractions such as the state, are the true actors and possess agency.[2] FPA theories at the individual, group, state-society, and international levels of analysis help focus theoretical attention and provide questions. They ask what factors influence or bear upon the individual actor or group of actors when deciding on a specific policy or course of action. For example, at the systemic level of analysis, FPA theory would lead us to inquire about the influence of the nature of the international system on individuals and groups of individuals by asking how perceptions of the international system (e.g., American primacy in the unipolar international system in the post–Cold War period) have influenced the actual policies adopted or pursued by various individuals. In other words, FPA theory would urge us to probe how precisely structural factors at the systemic level influence individuals or groups of individuals.[3] At the state-society level of analysis, this would also entail examination of how the political system (e.g., oligarchic system) or how ideational factors (e.g., ideology or religious beliefs) influence the foreign policies of individuals and groups of individuals. At the same time, as we shall see, mainstream FPA theory may be less than helpful in the Iranian case. Specifically, as concerns the role of religious ideology, I will argue that there is a real sense of boundedness that must be overcome to successfully apply FPA theory to the Iranian case.[4]

Realists posit the state to be a unitary rational actor, and thus they do not possess the theoretical capability to analyze the role of factions or religion or ideology in international relations.[5] According to Ole Holsti, when their theories do not explain what obviously has a basis in domestic politics, classical realists (in contrast to structural realists) "use domestic politics as a residual category to explain deviations from rational policies."[6] Realists—even the neoclassical realists, the branch of realism most suited for FPA—are skeptical toward the saliency and relevance of ideological goals as determinants of foreign policy.[7] For realists, material interests of the state, and not religious and ideological attributes of policymakers or the nature of the state, determine foreign policy.

Idealists do possess the theoretical capability to analyze ideational variables but tend to neglect religion or interpretations of religion as independent variable. Though FPA's middle-range theories are well suited to account for the role of ideational variables, emphasis is on culture and secular ideology, and the role of religion or religious ideology is neglected within mainstream FPA. This is probably due to the principle of separation of church and state enshrined in the U.S. political system.[8] Perhaps it is also due to the philosophical and intellectual roots of idealism which have been in the European enlightenment liberal thinkers, a tradition which was based on secularism, individualism, constitutionalism, tolerance, and capitalism, concepts and values that have been weak or absent in the Islamic tradition.[9] G. John Ikenberry, working within the idealist/liberal school of international relations, has demonstrated how America's liberal ideology has influenced America's grand strategy.[10] FPA theory of U.S. origin thus offers little to the analyst studying a country such as Iran, where religious ideology is paramount. Since 9/11, however, some FPA scholars have attempted to remedy that shortcoming.[11]

FPA theories do contain ideational theories of culture and (secular) ideology, but they seldom take religion and religious ideology seriously as an independent variable. Specifically, the role of Islamic fundamentalist ideology as a driver of foreign policy decision making is vastly underdeveloped.[12] This is surprising considering that the dominant paradigm in the study of the Middle East and Islamic fundamentalism is the "Islamic Exceptionalism" paradigm, which attributes the status of a causal independent variable to Islam.[13] For these scholars, Islam determines the behavior of the rulers and the ruled alike. This article illustrates that various factions of the ruling fundamentalist elites in Iran have divergent foreign policy behaviors; therefore, one could not say that Islam (or Shia Islam) is the independent variable determining the foreign policy behavior of various factions and individuals. Rather, each faction has its own interpretations of Shia Islam and fundamentalist ideology, which in turn have been transformed to distinct ideological and policy platforms. Thereupon, interpretations of Shia Islam and Islamic fundamentalist ideology act as causal factors. In other words, ahistorical Islam and ahistorical Shia Islam are not independent variables, but their interpretations appear to be so.

Religious ideology in general and Islamic fundamentalist ideologies are different than secular ideologies. They certainly are vastly different than liberal ideologies that dominate the liberal-idealist theories within FPA. Many variants of Islamic fundamentalist ideologies oppose the Westphalian state system, not from a Marxian post-nationalist vantage point, but from a premodern, pre-Westphalian Islamic point of view that wants to reestablish the Islamic *ummah* (*velayat* in Shia Islam and caliphate in Sunni Islam). For example, the Lebanese Hezbollah considers its supreme leader to be Ayatollah Khamenei, and before him it was Ayatollah Khomeini. This means that the Lebanese Hezbollah will go to war when it is ordered to so do by the supreme leader of Iran, and not the president of Lebanon.[14] Iran has been trying to establish similar groups in Iraq (e.g., Kataib Hezbollah, Supreme Council for Islamic Revolution in Iraq, and Badr Brigade), Saudi Arabia (e.g., Hezbollah al-Hijaz) and other Shia-populated areas.[15]

Much of the literature on Iranian foreign policy decision making presents a dichotomy of Iranian foreign policy to be either "rational and pragmatic" or "irrational and ideological."[16] This study presents a more nuanced analysis on the question of religious, ideological, and rational elements of Iranian foreign policy decision making.

Possibly due to its American origins, conventional FPA theory posits a straightforward correspondence between ideology (e.g., religion) and preferred policy outcomes.[17] Unfortunately, this assumption is not correct, and the Iranian case shows this clearly. First, this article will show that different factions and factional leaders hold divergent interpretations of Islam as their ideologies and notions of pragmatic cost-benefit analysis. So, some factions and leaders promote and pursue pragmatic and rational foreign policies based upon cost-benefit analyses, while others promote and pursue religiously derived ideological foreign policies. Second, this study also distinguishes between means and goals. For some leaders and sub-factions, foreign policy objectives are ideological, but many short-term means may be based on pragmatic and realistic methods.

Religious rationality is different than secular rationality. According to Holsti, classical realists assume that

> the states are guided by the logic of the "national interest," usually defined in terms of survival, security, power, and relative capabilities. To Morgenthau, for example, "rational foreign policy minimizes risks and maximizes benefits." Although the national interest may vary according to specific circumstances, the similarity of motives among nations permits the analyst to reconstruct the logic of policymakers in their pursuit of national interests—what Morgenthau called the "rational hypothesis"—and to avoid the fallacies of "concern with motives and concern with ideological preferences."[18]

Khamenei's foreign policy goals are ideological, such as opposing the current international system as well as confronting the U.S. and Israel. These polices have been the actual policies of Iran under both Khomeini and Khamenei, and Iran has paid a very high price for pursuing them. In response to other fundamentalists who have been pressuring Khamenei to back down to pressure from the U.S., Khamenei has said: "If the enemy puts a lot of pressure here, what happened in Karbala will happen here."[19] In Karbala, the Third Shia Imam Hussein fought a battle in which he and all his male supporters were killed by the Sunnis. In this context, Khamenei is saying that he is willing to engage is a mass suicidal war against the United States. Khamenei's privately stated policy does not conform to a secular rational policy. However, both these goals and means are consistent with the fundamentalist Shia ideology as well as with Shia theological beliefs.[20]

The oligarchical nature of the Iranian regime

Iran is not a one-man dictatorship. Rather, it is ruled by an oligarchy composed of fundamentalist clerics and laypersons. The Iranian oligarchy is not, and has never been, very cohesive. It is divided by social class, policy preferences, and individual ambition for power. The relative power of various individuals and factions has fluctuated since the Islamic Revolution in 1979. In order to understand Iranian foreign policy, it is therefore essential to understand the policies of the top members of the oligarchy and their factions.

The constitution and the political institutions in Iran are not epiphenomena. Rather, the constitutional rules and powers do matter in the intra-elite struggles in the short term. However, the constitutional rules and the institutions are not as significant in Iran as they are in advanced democracies. Part of the struggle among members of the oligarchy revolves around who should occupy which position of power in various institutions and how much power each institution should have. The power of various institutions and positions are spelled out by the constitution and by the various institutions' bylaws. Due to power struggles, the actual powers of various positions and institutions have evolved greatly since 1979. Therefore, it is essential to understand the de jure and de facto roles of various institutions.

This article presents a discussion on constitutional powers pertaining to foreign policy in Iran. Next, the policies of various factions, sub-factions, and individuals on foreign policy are described. Finally, the study analyzes how the constitutional powers and factional politics have played out, shaped, and determined Iran's foreign policy in the case of the nuclear issue.

The Iranian constitution and foreign policy

The roles and powers of various institutions are outlined in the constitution.[21] The constitution the fundamentalists wrote in 1979 included many flaws which exacerbated the intra-elite struggles. For example, it created the institutions of president and prime minister but was not clear on who makes foreign policy. By 1988, it became clear that serious changes had to be made before Supreme Leader Ruhollah

Khomeini's death. Many major changes were made in the 1989 revised constitution in order to streamline decision making and resolve some of the conflicts while preserving the power bases of various powerful elites.

To begin with, the position of prime minister was eliminated and its powers transferred to that of the president. Moreover, two new bodies were created: the Council for the Expediency of the System (Expediency Council) and the Supreme National Security Council (SNSC). The Expediency Council was created already in 1988 and was intended to resolve the differences between the *Majles* (parliament) and the Council of Guardians (a twelve-member body that, among other powers, can review the decisions of the *Majles* for compatibility with Sharia and the constitution) on domestic issues. The Expediency Council was subsequently added in the 1989 revised constitution and was to also provide the consensus of the elites on major issues to the supreme leader, especially regarding long-term grand strategies on economic and foreign policies. In turn, the SNSC was supposed to create consensus on specific short-term issues on foreign policy, national security, defense, and domestic security. Although not in the constitution, a new office emerged entitled "Office of the Supreme Leader" (OSL). The OSL has gradually become powerful, as discussed in greater detail below. Yet, its power is vicarious and depends on the supreme leader.

Iran's political system is called *Nezam Velayat Faghih* ("System of Rule by a High-Ranking Shia Clergy"). No one person fully controls *Nezam* ("the system"). The constitution has given executive, legislative, and judicial powers to the supreme leader (a high-ranking Shia cleric), but it also created the powerful Council of Guardians as well as an elected president, an elected *Majles*, and an elected Assembly of Experts. The Council of Guardians decides who can, or cannot, run for elected offices and allows only loyal fundamentalists to contest office. Although Supreme Leader Ali Khamenei, who assumed this position after Khomeini's death in 1989, is the most powerful official, he could be eased out of power if a majority of the members of the oligarchy so wish. The Assembly of Experts, which usually meets once a year, has the constitutional power to supervise, remove, and select the supreme leader.

The Ministry of Foreign Affairs and the foreign minister

The Ministry of Foreign Affairs, which is headed by the foreign minister, conducts the routine and mundane issues related to foreign policy. The constitution explicitly states that the foreign minister is nominated by the president, and has to be confirmed by the *Majles*. According to the constitution, the president can dismiss the members of the cabinet, including the foreign minister. At the same time, the constitution stipulates that the supreme leader is the ultimate power in foreign policy. It is not clear in practice whether the foreign minister answers to the president or the supreme leader.

The exact nature of that relationship among the foreign minister, president, and the supreme leader is dynamic and depends on the power balance between the supreme leader and the president. Who the foreign minister is and to whom he answers constitutes a significant aspect of the intra-elite struggles. While a player, the foreign minister is not the most powerful actor in foreign policy decision making in Iran.

The president

According to the constitution, the president is the head of the executive branch. However, the constitution also grants the supreme leader a great deal of executive power. The de facto powers of the presidency have waxed and waned since 1989. Between 1989 and 1997, under the presidency of Ali Akbar Hashemi Rafsanjani, the president made almost all the major decisions on foreign policy. Between 1997 and 2005, under the presidency of Mohammad Khatami, the supreme leader was in conflict with the president and attempted to undermine him at various junctures with mixed results.

Between 2005 and early 2011, when Khamenei agreed with president Ahmadinejad's policies, the latter was given a wide latitude to conduct foreign policy. Behind the scenes and occasionally publicly, the supreme leader provided great support to Ahmadinejad.[22] During this period, Ahmadinejad was able to fully utilize the powers that the constitution provides the presidency. This changed when conflict between Khamenei and Ahmadinejad became public. The conflict concerned the control over the activities of the foreign minister and the minister of intelligence. In December 2010, Ahmadinejad unilaterally dismissed foreign minister Manochehr Mottaki (a pragmatic hard-liner). When Ahmadinejad decided in April 2011 to also unilaterally dismiss Heydar Moslehi, the minister of intelligence (a hard-liner close to Khamenei), the supreme leader announced that he had reinstated the minister. According to the letter of the constitution, the president had the power to dismiss the members of his cabinet. However, within eleven days it became clear that actual power resided in the hands of the supreme leader, and the president had to either resign or submit to the supreme leader's demands. Many hard-liners wanted to dismiss Ahmadinejad, but Khamenei wanted him to remain in office, albeit with little power and fully submissive to him. Ahmadinejad complied and fully submitted to the supreme leader. Consequently, after April 2011 Ahmadinejad did not have much power, even that granted to the presidency by the constitution. Ahmadinejad's role in foreign policy was then eclipsed by foreign minister Ali Akbar Salehi (a pragmatic hard-liner) and the secretary of the SNSC, Saeed Jalili (an ultra-hard-liner close to the supreme leader).

When Hassan Rouhani became president in 2013, the office of the president had already lost a great amount of power to the office of the supreme leader. Rouhani's ability to pursue his foreign policy goals (e.g., nuclear negotiations with world powers to limit Iran's nuclear program in exchange for lifting of sanctions) has been dependent on his ability to persuade Khamenei to allow him to do so.[23]

It is widely believed that an arrangement has emerged between the president and the supreme leader that for several sensitive cabinet posts, the president has to get the consent of the supreme leader before he submits his nominations to the *Majles*. These are: foreign minister, defense minister, minister of intelligence, interior minister (a powerful position which oversees elections, appoints governors and deputy governors of the provinces, as well as coordinates with the police over security), and minister of culture and Islamic guidance.[24] Sometimes the negotiations may be long; Dorri Najafabadi was reportedly the fourteenth person that Khatami had suggested for the post of minister of intelligence.[25]

Supreme National Security Council

The purpose of the SNSC is to help establish consensus among the elites on various issues related to foreign policy, national security, defense, and domestic security. The supreme leader appoints two members; other members include the president, the foreign minister, the minister of defense, the minister of intelligence, the minister of the interior, the chairman of the joint chiefs, the commander of the Islamic Revolutionary Guards Corps (IRGC), the head of the judicial branch, and the speaker of the *Majles*, among others. While the president heads the SNSC, the secretary of the SNSC wields great power. All the decisions of the SNSC are submitted to the supreme leader for approval. After the supreme leader approves them, they become the official policy of Iran. Those policies are then sent to various ministries or departments for implementation.[26]

The secretaries of the SNSC have been Hassan Rouhani (October 1989 to August 2005), Ali Larijani (August 2005 to October 2007), Saeed Jalili (October 2007 to September 2013), and IRGC Admiral Ali Shamkhani (September 2013 to present). All the secretaries of the SNSC have been one of the two appointees of the supreme leader. Although the president appoints the secretary of the SNSC, which is not a cabinet position and does not require *Majles* confirmation, it is widely believed that he should get the consent of the supreme leader before making the appointment.[27]

Supreme leader

According to the constitution, the supreme leader has the ultimate authority on foreign policy, defense, national security, war, and peace. He is the head of all the armed forces and coercive apparatuses: the IRGC, *Basij* (a "volunteer" paramilitary entity used to attack domestic opponents of the regime and mobilize the youth for the war effort against foreign foes, which is now a section of the IRGC), regular armed forces, and the police. At the same time, the constitution grants actual powers to various other institutions and offices as indicated in the preceding paragraphs.

While Khomeini was alive, his words were accepted by all the members of the oligarchy. Between 1989 and 1997, actual power was exercised by President Rafsanjani, and the new Supreme Leader Khamenei stayed out of his way. They would meet once a week, when Rafsanjani would inform the supreme leader of various policies. Khamenei simply approved all the decisions that were made by the Expediency Council and the SNSC. The sole issue that the supreme leader insisted upon was that no rapprochement with the U.S. was allowed. On all other issues (foreign and domestic), Khamenei simply followed the lead of Rafsanjani and the consensus of the elites forwarded to him by the Expediency Council and the SNSC.[28] Since 1997, the supreme leader has pushed back the influence of the president and reasserted the institution's dominant position on foreign policy.

Intra-elite factionalism and foreign policy

There are three main factions among the fundamentalists: expedients, reformists, and hard-liners. Each faction comprises several sub-factions. The leadership and composition of the factions have remained relatively stable. At certain junctures, various sub-factions have made alliances with other factions rather than with their own faction.[29] For example, on several occasions, some hard-liners such as Ali Larijani (speaker of the *Majles*, secretary of SNSC, and presidential candidate), Ali Akbar Nategh-Nouri (presidential candidate in 1997 and senior adviser to the supreme leader at OSL), and Ali Mottahari (maverick and powerful member of the *Majles* and son of the late Ayatollah Morteza Mottahari, who was the main fundamentalist theoretician of the revolution) worked with Rafsanjani to undermine Ahmadinejad. The above-mentioned pragmatic hard-liners have provided crucial support to Rouhani since he became president.

The primary foreign policy issues dividing the oligarchy revolve around relations with the U.S., assistance to radical groups, the Israel-Palestinian conflict, regional influence, and the nuclear program. All factions wish to preserve fundamentalist rule but disagree on the policies which would best serve that end.

Expedients

The expedient faction, led by Rafsanjani, proposes what is called the "Chinese model": détente with the U.S., entente with the European Union (EU), close cooperation with Russia and China, increased political repression, and laxer enforcement of social restrictions such as those on music and Islamic dress for women.[30] The expedients strongly fear the consequences of economic sanctions and believe that behind-the-scenes deals with the U.S. could resolve the conflict.[31] They also believe that economic improvement and reduction of social restrictions would coopt enough of the population (especially educated urban technocrats) to secure the regime. The Executives of Construction Party reflects the views of this faction.

Rafsanjani has been one of the most powerful officials in Iran since the 1979 revolution. He has served as speaker of the *Majles* (1980–1989), acting commander of the armed forces during the Iran–Iraq war (Khomeini had transferred his powers to him), president (1989–1997), and chairman of the Assembly of Experts. He has been head of the Expediency Council since 1989 (when it was established) and a member of the Assembly of Experts. He is widely regarded as one of the richest and most corrupt officials, although he denies the charges. In the early 1990s, with help from the supreme leader and other hard-liners, Rafsanjani purged the "Left Fundamentalists" (who became the reformists by 1997) from various positions of power. Because of this, many reformists have had a hard time forgiving Rafsanjani for purging them.[32] Rafsanjani opposes policies that could provoke a war with the U.S. Rafsanjani argues that direct negotiations with the U.S. could resolve the crisis. He has been gathering support among the elites to change the policies pursued by the ultra-hard-liners. He succeeded by helping Rouhani, who has been one of the most authoritarian and conservative members of the expedient faction, become president in 2013.[33] Members of the lists supported by Rafsanjani gained seats for the Assembly of Experts and the *Majles* in the February 2016 elections. Rafsanjani himself received the highest number of votes for the Assembly of Experts.

Reformists

Between 1979 and the early 1990s, the left fundamentalists were the most extremist, violent, antidemocratic, and anti-American members of the ruling oligarchy. The overwhelming majority of the leaders of the fundamentalist students, called "Students Followers of the Imam [Khomeini's] Line," who attacked the U.S. embassy and held Americans at the embassy hostage for 444 days, were left fundamentalists. The main leaders of this faction were Ayatollah Sadegh Khalkhali (the head of the revolutionary courts, known in the West as the "hanging judge"), Ayatollah Mohammad Moussavi Khoeiniha (the leader of the fundamentalist students who took over the American embassy and their liaison with Ayatollah Khomeini), Hojatolislam Ali Akbar Mohtashami-pour (minister of interior and ambassador to Syria who helped found the Lebanese Hezbollah), Hojatolislam Hadi Ghafari (one of the most extreme, violent, and authoritarian members of the oligarchy), Mir Hussein Moussavi, Mehdi Karrubi, and Mohammad Khatami.

The left fundamentalists dominated the *Majles* until 1992.[34] Many of them advocated that Iran side with Saddam Hussein in the 1991 war between the U.S. and Iraq.[35] During their purge from power (1992–1997), they transformed themselves from left fundamentalists to reformist members of the oligarchy. Once they were purged from the positions of power, the left fundamentalists began a process of serious analysis on the failures of the system. Being expelled from the positions of power made them antagonistic toward the authoritarian features of the system. The left fundamentalists promoted statist economic policies. The collapse of communism in the former USSR and Eastern Europe, as well as capitalist economic reorientation in China, made the left fundamentalists realize that prosperity could not be achieved through statist economics. They also believed that the post–Cold War period is a unipolar system with American primacy; therefore, picking fights with the U.S. could cause great harm to the regime. One of the major issues in the 1990s and early 2000s was democratization. So, whereas in 1979 the left fundamentalists were very hostile to the liberal democrats in the provisional government (for promoting good relations with the U.S., democracy, moderation, and mixed economy), by 1997–present, the now-reformists came to realize that some liberal democratic policies make sense. Moreover, in the 1990s, the U.S. had become very popular among the Iranian people, especially the urban middle classes who were suffering under the Islamic Republic's economic mismanagement, political repression, and cultural suffocation. Reformist members of the oligarchy concluded that by promoting a reduction of restrictions on the press, they could communicate with the people. By promoting competitive elections (among fundamentalists) they could come back to positions of power if they reflected the wishes of the people who were craving economic prosperity, political freedoms, and cultural openness. The reformists are not democrats. They support the antidemocratic fundamentalist constitution and the system of *Velayat Faghih*. The reformists do not advocate replacement of the ruling theocracy with democracy, nor do they advocate allowing pro-democracy political parties the right to participate in elections. They want to make reforms in order to preserve the Islamic Republic.

The reformist faction returned to power during the presidency of Mohammad Khatami (1997–2005). They also controlled the *Majles* between 2000 and 2004. However, the hard-liners succeeded in pushing out the reformists from the city councils in 2003, the *Majles* in 2004, and the presidency in 2005. In the aftermath of the 2009 presidential elections, the hard-liners utterly crushed the reformists, placing many of their leaders in prison (e.g., Mohsen Aminzadeh, deputy foreign minister during Khatami's presidency, who is the most articulate theoretician of the reformist faction on foreign policy) or under house arrest (Moussavi and Karrubi).

Reformists have reached the conclusion that the post–Cold War period is a unipolar system with American primacy. Their primary foreign policy goals are avoiding wars, stabilizing domestic politics, and pursuing economic prosperity. To accomplish those goals, they argue that the regime should abandon ideologically driven foreign policies and instead pursue national interests as the goals of foreign policy utilizing rational and pragmatic means. These policies are designed to resolve the domestic crisis of legitimacy and to improve the international image of the regime. More specifically, the reformists advocate expanding the number of allies, transforming neutrals into friends, rivals into neutrals, and enemies into rivals. Fearing an American military invasion and economic sanctions, reformists propose to improve relations with the U.S. Moreover, they want to reach an entente with the EU and Iran's neighbors (especially Saudi Arabia and Turkey), maintain good relations with Russia and China, suspend uranium enrichment, and reduce political repression and social restrictions at home.[36] Indeed, during his presidency Khatami succeeded in transforming Saudi Arabia from an enemy to a rival or even friend. He also succeeded in improving the relations with the EU, several Arab countries, and Turkey.[37] Overall, the reformists want to have as few enemies as possible, and do not want to provoke them. They criticize the hard-liners for doing the opposite: turning friends into neutrals, neutrals into rivals, rivals into enemies, and expanding the number of enemies and unnecessarily provoking them.

Hard-liners

Khomeini's failure between 1979 and 1989 to overthrow the regimes in Iraq, Saudi Arabia, Lebanon, Egypt, and Bahrain, as well as the terrible cost of the war with Iraq, compelled many in the ruling fundamentalist oligarchy, such as Rafsanjani and Khatami, to suspend such aggressive policies, and instead concentrate on rebuilding the Iranian economy. However, the rise of Ahmadinejad in 2005 and the support given to him by Khamenei between 2005 and mid-2011 resulted in a return to the bellicose policies of Khomeini. The rise of ultra-hard-line groups indicates the emergence of ultra-hawkish and ultra-bellicose elements in Iran's oligarchy.

The hard-liners, led by the supreme leader, believe that departure from the early ideals and policies of the revolution under the presidencies of Rafsanjani (1989–1997) and Khatami (1997–2005) are the causes of the crisis. They advocate the export of the radical Islamic fundamentalist revolution, increased conflict with the U.S. and Israel, increased political repression (e.g., imprisonment of political dissenters, violence against women activists, and purging of nonfundamentalist university students and professors), stricter imposition of Islamic rules, such as the ban of Western music, stricter enforcement of women's *hejab*, and harsher censorship of movies, books, newspapers, internet sites, and blogs. The hard-liners oppose the current international system. They believe that a handful of powerful countries, led by the U.S. and including the European powers, controls and plunders the world. Accordingly, hard-liners want to alter the current international system. They condemn the veto power that the five permanent members of the United Nations Security Council (UNSC) enjoy. They also want to abolish the state of Israel and make it illegal to insult, criticize, or undermine the beliefs of adherents of the Abrahamic religions, Judaism, Christianity, and Islam, the only faiths they regard as true faiths. They say that they want a radical redistribution of global wealth, although they do not specify exactly how this ought to be accomplished.[38]

Many hard-liners believe that the U.S. is engaged in psychological warfare and discount the possibility of any U.S. military action. They think that if the regime gave in on the nuclear issue, the U.S. would bring up other issues such as human rights, democracy, assistance to radical Islamist groups (Hezbollah, Hamas, and Palestinian Islamic Jihad), and recognition of Israel—issues in which the regime could lose its legitimacy among its supporters if it were to give in. Thus, they advocate taking their stand on the nuclear issue as one with the most support among the population.

The hard-line faction contains different tendencies in regard to foreign policy. These tendencies have not yet solidified into sub-factions. For lack of better terms, I use the following labels to describe these tendencies: pragmatic hard-liners; ultra-hard-liners opposed to talks and negotiations with the U.S.; hard-liners supportive of talks with the U.S.; messianic ultra-hard-liners opposed to negotiations with the U.S.; and messianic ultra-hard-liners supportive of negotiations with the U.S.

The pragmatic hard-liners (e.g., Ali Larijani and Generals Mohsen Rezaee and Mohammad Bagher Ghalibaf) are fully subservient to the supreme leader but want to avoid war with the U.S. Larijani, Rezaee (former commander-in-chief of the IRGC and frequent candidate for president), and Ghalibaf (former commander of IRGC Air Force, former head of police, mayor of Tehran, and candidate for president in 2005 and 2013) have publicly advocated détente with the outside world in mid- to late 2012.[39] The pragmatic hard-liners use cost-benefit analysis in reaching their decisions. In 2005, they supported reneging on the concessions made by Iran on the nuclear program in 2003–2004. In 2005, the U.S. appeared to be facing serious difficulties in Iraq and Afghanistan and thus was unable to use military means to impose its will on Iran. In their view, due to the world's need for Iranian oil, serious crippling sanctions were considered unlikely. However, as the likelihood of military strikes and serious economic sanctions grew during 2012 and 2013, they began to support making concessions on the nuclear program.[40]

A powerful group of ultra-hard-liners (e.g., Ahmad Jennati, chairman of the Council of Guardians and a member of the Assembly of Experts, Ayatollah Mesbah Yazdi, Saeed Jalili, Hussein Shariatmadari, Ali Reza Zakani, and Hamid Rasaee) opposes any negotiations with the U.S. as a matter of ideology and policy. For this group, the U.S. should be confronted as a matter of principle, rather than based on a cost-benefit analysis. This tendency advocates more bellicose policies toward the U.S. and the EU. They do not fear military conflict with the West; rather, they seem to welcome it, since they believe that Iran would win any such confrontation. They also advocate more hostile and belligerent policies toward pro-American governments in the region, such as those in Saudi Arabia and Jordan. They opposed rapprochement with the Mubarak regime in Egypt during Khatami's presidency. They regard the overthrow of Hosni Mubarak of Egypt and Ben Ali of Tunisia as vindication of their views and policies.[41] Members of this group strongly oppose the Joint Comprehensive Program of Action (JCPOA), the agreement reached between Iran and the P5+1 on July 14, 2015. According to the JCPOA, sanctions imposed on Iran due to its nuclear program would be lifted in exchange for Iran dismantling key aspects of its nuclear program, such as modifying the heavy water plant in Arak, warehousing most of its centrifuges, transferring its enriched uranium and heavy water to other countries, modifying the underground uranium enrichment facility at Fordo, answering IAEA's questions on unresolved possible military dimensions of the program, and allowing more inspections of suspected facilities.[42] Members of this group in the *Majles*, led by Zakani and Rasaee, opposed the passage of the deal. Several prominent members of this group lost their seats for the *Majles* and the Assembly of Experts in the February 2016 elections. Both Zakani and Rasaee lost their *Majles* seats. Ayatollah Mesbah lost his seat at the Assembly of Experts.

Conversely, some other hard-liners (above all Khamenei) do not oppose talks with the U.S. as a matter of principle. These hard-liners support "topical talks" with the U.S. on issues such as Afghanistan, Iraq, or drug trafficking, or multilateral talks which include the U.S., such as those conducted under the aegis of the P5+1 (permanent members of the UNSC plus Germany) over the nuclear issue. However, their position on the sensitive notion of "comprehensive negotiations" with the U.S. to resolve the conflicts between the two countries has not been consistent. At some junctures, Khamenei has absolutely opposed such comprehensive negotiations due to what he considers to be the natures of the U.S. and Iran. However, at other junctures, he has said that he might decide to have such negotiations under certain conditions.[43] Khamenei and those in this tendency believe that the U.S. is too weak to impose its will on Iran. Khamenei prefers to contain American power in the region, while others believe a roll-back of American hegemony is possible. Khamenei has been pursuing a policy of stalling and buying time.

Khamenei considers the primary struggle in the post–Cold War period to be between the U.S. and Iran. He considers the U.S. to be leading a bloc of countries that promotes the current international system based on liberal democracy, secularism, capitalism, and American domination of the world. He regards Iran to be spearheading the bloc challenging the current system. He promotes Islamic fundamentalism, struggle against Israel, and assistance to radical militant groups. Khamenei also believes that liberal democracy, secularism, and American hegemony are in decline. Still, he wishes to avoid any direct military confrontation with the U.S. or with Israel, at least for the time being. Khamenei is against rapprochement with the U.S. He fears that comprehensive negotiations might create more harm than benefit. He believes that a policy of containment of the U.S. in the region via gradual bleeding by proxies such as the Lebanese Hezbollah, Moqtada al-Sadr's Jeish al-Mahdi, Asaib Ahl al-Haq (League of the Righteous), and Kataib Hezbollah (Hezbollah Brigades) in Iraq, as well as various groups in Afghanistan, would cause the Americans to withdraw from the region. Khamenei has argued that militant Islamic fundamentalist groups have been and will be on the rise in Egypt, Yemen, Bahrain, Libya, Algeria, Jordan, and Turkey, among many others.[44] This faction includes powerful figures such as Ayatollah Ahmad Khatami (member of the Assembly of Experts and no relationship with former president Mohammad Khatami), Ayatollah Mohammad Yazdi (former chairman of the Assembly of Experts until he lost his seat in the February 2016 election), and Ayatollah Ahmad Alamolhoda (member of the Assembly of Experts).

The most extremist and bellicose sub-faction is the ultra-hard-liners with messianic viewpoints who oppose negotiations with the U.S. Members holding this tendency believe that we live during the period of the reappearance of the twelfth Imam Mahdi, the Shia messiah.[45] In Iran they are called "*mo'aod-gara*" (messianic or apocalyptic). The supreme leader directly controls the IRGC through appointing the *Namayandeh Vali Faghih* (representative of the supreme leader) to the IRGC. These are clerics who are situated at the very top of the IRGC, but also within the entire corps. The top representative of the supreme leader to the IRGC is Hojatolislam Valialmoslemin Ali Saeedi. Saeedi argues that the supreme leader, IRGC, and the IRGC's Qods Force will be playing the primary roles in the reappearance of the twelfth Imam.[46] He also strongly opposes any negotiations with the U.S.

Finally, there is a group of messianic ultra-hard-liners who support negotiations with the U.S.[47] Ahmadinejad is the most prominent member of this sub-faction. At least since the election of President Obama, Ahmadinejad has publicly called for negotiation with the U.S. Unlike Khamenei, he thinks it might be possible and desirable to reach an understanding with the U.S.—including on the nuclear issue. Like Jennati, Ahmadinejad believes that in a military confrontation with the U.S., Iran will be victorious. Ahmadinejad believes that it is possible to hold negotiations with the U.S. and convince them to leave the region without a war. Although Ahmadinejad is far less hostile to the U.S. than Khamenei or Jennati, he uses more provocative language, especially with regard to the Holocaust and the 9/11 attacks. Many in this group want Iran to be a nuclear threshold state, and argue that the Rouhani administration has given too many concessions to the U.S. and P5+1. The daily *Vatan Emruz*, which is run by Ahmadinejad's former officials and supporters, called the Joint Plan of Action, the temporary agreement reached between the Rouhani government and the P5+1, the "nuclear Holocaust."[48] This group remains hostile to the JCPOA.

Between mid-2011 and the end of Ahmadinejad's tenure, foreign policy decisions were made by the supreme leader with inputs from OSL advisors (Velayati and Safavi), former foreign minister Salehi (who directly answered to him), and the former secretary of the SNSC, Jalili (who directly answered to him), the IRGC top commanders (Jafaari), and supreme leader's representative to the IRGC, Saeedi. The situation seemed to be an exception in the history of the Islamic Republic. For the first time, foreign policy was not made through reaching a consensus among the various factions of the fundamentalist elites; instead it was made by the supreme leader and a handful of his own advisers plus the top commanders of the IRGC. The IRGC has begun playing more prominent roles in foreign policy.[49] For example, it is believed that the portfolio for Iraq was taken from the foreign minister and the president and given to the IRGC.[50] The IRGC also has a major say on the nuclear program, much of which is conducted under its supervision and command.[51] The supreme commander of the IRGC is Gen. Mohammad Ali Jafaari.

However, the devastating sanctions that went into effect in the summer of 2012 appeared to threaten the stability of the regime, thus compelling Khamenei to allow Rouhani to become president in order to counter the threat of sanctions. Allowing Rouhani to become president resulted in an increase in the power of the expedient faction and a reduction of the power of ultra-hard-liners close to Ayatollah Mesbah. Khamenei's power, although still great, has been reduced slightly since mid-2013. Khamenei's retreat since 2013, the election of Rouhani in 2013, the February 2016 elections, and the JCPOA have consolidated the regime and have greatly helped the regime overcome the crises due to the 2009 mass protests and the economic downturn due to the sanctions. Khamenei's retreat (what he termed "heroic flexibility") on the nuclear program constituted allowing Rouhani and his team (e.g., Mohammad Javad Zarif the foreign minister) to make concessions in exchange for lifting of the sanctions. Rouhani was able to gain the upper hand against the ultra-hard-liners in the intra-elite struggles by allying with the reformists by promising them social, political, and economic reforms. For Khamenei (and hard-liners and pragmatic hard-liners), Rouhani is useful to the extent that he succeeds in removing the sanctions and improves the economy, and becomes harmful to the extent that he succeeds in the political and social reforms as well as other foreign policy areas (e.g., détente with the U.S., regional policies toward Saudi Arabia, Iraq, Syria, Lebanon, Yemen, and Israel). Khamenei wants Rouhani to only engage and succeed in the nuclear agreement and sanctions removal.[52] Khamenei has the power to undermine Rouhani's activities in other foreign policy arenas as well as on social, economic, and political realms, although they will come at a steep cost to the stability of the regime if Rouhani or his reformist and expedient allies were to mobilize and protest publicly, as occurred after the disputed 2009 elections. In order to restrain Rouhani while not undermining the JCPOA and sanctions removal, Khamenei and the hard-liners have taken a number of actions, such as testing a ballistic missile (with the slogan "Israel must be wiped off the face of the earth" in Hebrew and Persian on the missile),[53] broadcasting films of underground missile cities and silos,[54] shooting rockets around 1,500 yards from an American aircraft carrier in the Persian Gulf by the IRGC Navy,[55] broadcasting the humiliating treatment of American Navy personnel who were detained after they had veered into Iranian territorial waters,[56] clandestinely shipping large amounts of weapons to Yemen,[57] arresting Iranian-American dual citizens, dramatically increasing executions,[58] jailing of Rafsanjani's son on corruption charges, and continuing to keep Moussavi and Karrubi under house arrest (their release was among Rouhani's campaign promises). Expedients (particularly Rafsanjani) and reformists will pressure Rouhani to stand up to Khamenei and to carry out his promises on foreign policy as well as economic, political, and social reforms. Thus, the situation remains highly volatile and dynamic due to a lack of consensus among the fundamentalist elites on major foreign policy concerns.

Case study: The Iranian nuclear program

In the mid-1980s, Iran started its clandestine nuclear program.[59] At the time, Iraq was using chemical weapons on Iranian troops as well SCUD missiles with conventional payloads to attack population centers in major cities. According to Shahram Chubin, one of the world's foremost authorities on Iran's nuclear program, Iran's program was a weapons program from the 1980s. In Chubin's words:

> Iran's nuclear program, initially cancelled after the 1979 revolution, was revived in the closing phases of the 1980–1988 war with Iraq. Tehran wanted to guard against a future surprise analogous to Iraq's repeated use of chemical weapons ....Iran appears to have wanted to start a secret program for several reasons, from its experience during Iran–Iraq War to the fact that five of the world's nine nuclear powers are nearby or on its borders. At the time, it also appears to have adopted a strategy of nuclear hedging—or maintaining the *option* of a weapons program, while trying to remain within the nuclear treaty ....Iran's nuclear weapons program was part of a broader attempt to become more self-reliant in arms and technology in the 1980s. Increasingly isolated, Tehran struggled to acquire arms to fight Iraq, which used chemical weapons and had a nuclear weapons program.[60]

According to the International Atomic Energy Agency (IAEA),

> Iran has carried out the following activities that are relevant to the development of a nuclear explosive devise ....The acquisition of nuclear weapons development information and documentation from a clandestine network ....Work on the development of an indigenous design of a nuclear weapon including the testing of components.[61] According to Takeyh, "the circumstantial evidence strongly suggests that Iran is, at a minimum, aiming to develop a nuclear weapons capability."[62] According to Haghighatjoo, a prominent reformist and former member of the *Majles* who now lives in the U.S., powerful hard-liners supported the development of nuclear weapons.[63]

Between 1986 and 2003, Iran's clandestine nuclear weapons program was directed, pursued, and implemented by *all* the ruling factions (expedient, reformist, and hard-line). According to A. Q. Khan (the father of Pakistan's nuclear bomb who confessed to having sold know-how and materials to Iran and Libya), Ali Shamkhani (one of the founders of the IRGC, supreme commander of IRGC Navy, and minister of defense under Khatami) had gone to Pakistan to collect three finished nuclear bombs from Pakistan in 1987. Shamkhani's trip to Pakistan began the clandestine cooperation between Iran and Khan's network. Iran had offered a deal worth almost $10 billion.[64] Shamkhani (close to Rafsanjani and Rouhani) is currently the secretary of the SNSC. The Atomic Energy Organization of Iran (AEOI) is the civilian organization that has served as the cover for the clandestine nuclear weapons program, which is under the control of the IRGC. Between 1981 and 1997 its director was Reza Amrollahi and between 1997 and 2009 its director was Gholam Reza Aghazadeh. Amrollahi is a high-ranking member of the expedient faction and Aghazadeh is a reformist who resigned in 2009 in protest to the crackdown on the reformists. According to Rouhani, Iran's clandestine nuclear program activities were drastically increased between 1999 and 2002.[65] These are the years that the reformists and expedients controlled the presidency, SNSC,

AEOI, Expediency Council, and *Majles* (between 2000 and 2004), as well as a segment of the Assembly of Experts.

In November 2003, Iran agreed to temporarily suspend uranium enrichment and then signed the additional protocols allowing intrusive inspections by the IAEA.[66] This compromise was brokered by the EU3 (the UK, France, and Germany). The EU3 agreed to help prevent Iran's case to be referred from the IAEA to the UNSC in exchange for the agreements. Between mid-2005 and February 2006, Iran began rejecting a number of earlier agreements, such as the suspension of uranium enrichment and the implementation of additional protocols.[67] These caused Iran's case to be referred from the IAEA to the Security Council. Subsequently, Iran's refusal to abide by demands of the UNSC resulted in a number of Security Council resolutions imposing sanctions on Iran. Between 2013 and 2015, Iran agreed to make concessions on its nuclear program in exchange for removal of sanctions. What explains the dramatic change in Iran's nuclear policy?

In 2003, reformist Khatami was president and expedient Rouhani was the secretary of the SNSC. The reformist and expedient members of the oligarchy dominated the various foreign policy decision-making apparatuses and positions, such as foreign minister, deputy foreign minister, presidency, SNSC, and secretary of SNSC. Moreover, the reformists controlled the *Majles*, and the Expediency Council under the control of Rafsanjani was a powerful body. On the other hand, Khamenei and the hard-liners held a minority of positions within the foreign policy decision-making apparatuses.

After President Bush declared Iran as part of the axis of evil in January 2002, and the military invasions in October 2001 and March 2003 which overthrew the regimes in Afghanistan and Iraq, respectively, there was a palpable concern among many members of the oligarchy that Iran could be next on the American regime-change agenda.[68] The sensitive talks and policies on the nuclear file were conducted by the SNSC's secretary, Rouhani. He came under harsh criticisms for the compromises made with the EU3 in 2003–2004 agreeing both to suspend uranium enrichment and to the additional protocols. Rouhani had the support of Khatami (and the reformists) and Rafsanjani (and the expedients) in making those concessions, but was heavily criticized by hard-liners in the state television and radio (under the control of the supreme leader).[69]

Mohsen Aminzadeh, the deputy foreign minister during the eight -year presidency of Khatami, argues that the goal of Khatami's nuclear policy was to gain the confidence of other actors, above all the Europeans, so that Iran could continue its nuclear program, including finishing the Bushehr nuclear power plant and subsequently establishing a pilot industrial nuclear facility as well as nuclear scientific research facilities.[70] Aminzadeh writes that in the continuation of this trend, it was expected that a deal would be reached eventually in which Iran for its part would provide necessary guarantees to develop only peaceful nuclear industries. In return, Iran was supposed to get sufficient guarantees from the international community for its national security and also see all sanctions abolished.[71]

Aminzadeh considers the referral of Iran's nuclear dossier from the IAEA to the UNSC under the presidency of Ahmadinejad to be one of the major foreign policy defeats of the Islamic Republic. He fully blames the defeat on the policies of the hard-liners.[72] In 2005, hard-liners such as Ahmadinejad harshly criticized those concessions and the "weak" policies of the reformists and expedients. Soon other ultra-hard-liners, such as Jennati, joined the criticisms. Jennati is probably the second most powerful member of the hard-line faction. In 2006, during a Friday sermon at the University of Tehran (where top members of the oligarchy discuss the main issues confronting the regime), he criticized the manner in which reformist and expedient officials had conducted the nuclear negotiations. In his opinion, Iran wasted two years by agreeing to stop its nuclear enrichment activities. He then proceeded to lend his support to the new policy of confronting the EU and restarting the nuclear enrichment.[73]

Although Khamenei was publicly silent between 2003 and 2004 on the concessions, he made harsh criticisms of the policies later on. In his major foreign policy speech in 2012, Khamenei said that when Iran retreated between 2003 and July 2005, the West would not allow Iran to have even three centrifuges, but after he stepped in and changed Iran's policy, Iran had eleven thousand centrifuges by mid-2012.[74]

After Ahmadinejad's election in 2005, Rouhani was replaced as secretary of the SNSC by pragmatic hard-liner Ali Larijani. And after Larijani's resignation, the ultra-hard-line Saeed Jalili became the secretary of SNSC. The new team composed of mostly hard-line and ultra-hard-line elements pursued a policy they called *siasat khareji tahajomi* (aggressive and offensive foreign policy). Thus, by late August 2005 all foreign policy decision making positions were in the hands of hard-line elements. Moreover, the hard-liners controlled all the other institutions except the Expediency Council. This allowed them to change Iran's foreign policy to their liking.

Even so, the reformists strongly opposed the new aggressive policies of the hard-liners. The Islamic Iran Participation Front, the main reformist party, prepared a detailed and harsh statement of the hard-line nuclear policy in March 2006. The statement was going to be published on the party's official website, when the party was told by the ministry of intelligence that if it released the statement, it would be confronted and the party would be abolished.[75] The full text of the statement was published only in October 2012. The statement argued:

> It is shocking that relevant officials make official statements that we are not afraid of sanctions and war ....Within a short period, they have taken the country toward such a crisis and are proud of it ....Worries about the destiny of our country and nation have made us to call upon the officials to think about the problems of the people instead of thinking about their ideological goals that could never materialize ....Without a doubt our officials have provided the pretext to the dominant foreign powers, and here one cannot blame the enemy for taking maximum use of these opportunities, because it is natural for the enemy to want to use such opportunities, and we should not provide such pretexts and opportunities for them ....We suggest that officially and explicitly the government announces and emphasizes that our policy is détente and peaceful coexistence. And instead of the current language of creating enemies and confrontations, the officials should use appropriate language ....Our experiences prove that if the current policies are insisted upon, either our country is headed toward a full-scale confrontation with a huge chunk of the world, or all of the sudden and in the worst conditions, we will surrender to the demands of the opponents, or after serious problems we will gradually retreat from our positions. All three end-results will harm the country and are against the national interests.[76]

Overall, Iran's policy on the nuclear issue illustrates how competing factions controlling the foreign policy decision-making apparatuses have determined Iran's foreign policy. Between 2003 and July 2005, the reformists and expedients held the majority of foreign policy decision-making positions. Khamenei acquiesced to the consensus of the majority in the SNSC. The election of Ahmadinejad in 2005 changed the balance of forces among the elites. The hard-liners then reversed the earlier concessions. The new aggressive policy between 2005 and 2012 promised to help Iran greatly expand its nuclear program and possibly achieve its goal. Despite greatly advancing the nuclear program, the regime did not succeed in completing nuclear weapons. By early 2013, many pragmatic hard-liners, fearful of economic collapse in 2013, sided with expedients, and helped push for Rouhani and supported him in his policies of making concessions on the nuclear program. Khamenei, again, acquiesced with great reluctance. His official letter of approval was conditional and left the door wide open for withdrawal.[77]

Conclusion

If the analysis in this article is correct, with a change in the balance of power among the factions, we should expect a change in Iran's foreign policy in general and its adherence to the JCPOA in particular. There does not exist a consensus among the fundamentalist elites on the JCPOA, relations with the U.S., or the regional policy. Moreover, there does not exist a stable equilibrium or balance among the factions. Most significantly, ultra-hard-liners and many hard-liners as well as the IRGC strongly oppose the JCPOA. These forces have engaged in a number of provocative actions to scuttle the agreement. Dire economic conditions forced some of the elites to acquiesce to the agreement. As the economic conditions change (e.g., removal of sanctions and return of Iran's frozen funds), the reasons for the concessions will be removed. This will lead to a reduction of relevancy and necessity of policies advocated by expedients and reformists. This will also enhance the power of those advocating nuclear breakout covertly under the JCPOA or overtly after the dismantling of the JCPOA as long as there is little fear of military strikes. Many believe that the death of Khamenei (born 1939) will dramatically increase the power of the IRGC.[78] If such scholars are right, considering that the IRGC strongly opposes the JCPOA, it would be reasonable to assume that Iran will then either pursue covert nuclear weaponization under the JCPOA or officially leave the agreement.

Acknowledgments

I thank Valerie M. Hudson and Klaus Brummer for their suggestions and critiques of earlier versions of this article. This article owes a great deal to their theoretical and analytical guidance. I also thank Kevjn Lim for his suggestions. I am solely responsible for any errors of fact or interpretation.

Notes

1. Valerie M. Hudson, "Foreign Policy Analysis: Actor-Specific Theory and the Ground of International Relations," *Foreign Policy Analysis*, vol.1 (2005): 1–30; Hudson, *Foreign Policy Analysis: Classic and Contemporary Theory* (Lanham, MD: Rowman and Littlefield, 2007); Hudson, "The History and Evolution of Foreign Policy Analysis," in Steve Smith, Amelia Hadfield, and Tim Dunne, eds., *Foreign Policy: Theories, Actors, Cases*, 2nd ed. (Oxford: Oxford University Press, 2012), 13–34; and Chris Alden and Amnon Aran, *Foreign Policy Analysis: New Approaches* (London: Routledge, 2012).
2. Hudson, *Foreign Policy Analysis*, 6.
3. Walter Carlsnaes, "Actors, Structures, and Foreign Policy Analysis," in Smith et al., eds. , *Foreign Policy: Theories, Actors, Cases*, 113–129.
4. For excellent discussions on the limits of the FPA theory and how to overcome some of these limitations, see Valerie Hudson, "Introduction to Foreign Policy Analysis Beyond North America" and Klaus Brummer, "Implications from FPA Scholarship Beyond North America for Mainstream FPA Theory," both in Valerie Hudson and Klaus Brummer, eds., *Foreign Policy Analysis Beyond North America* (Boulder, CO: Lynne Rienner, 2015).
5. Ole R. Holsti, "Models of International Relations and Foreign Policy," in G. John Ikenberry, ed., *American Foreign Policy: Theoretical Essays*, 5th ed. (New York: Pearson Longman, 2005), 14–40.
6. Ibid., 16.
7. William C. Wohlforth, "Realism and Foreign Policy," in Steve Smith et al., eds., *Foreign Policy*, 37, 52.
8. I owe this argument to Valerie Hudson's comment on an earlier version of this article.
9. Tim Dunne, "Liberalism," in John Baylis, Steve Smith, and Patricia Owens, eds., *The Globalization of World Politics: An Introduction to International Relations*, 6th ed. (Oxford: Oxford University Press, 2014), 114.
10. G. John Ikenberry, "America's Liberal Grand Strategy," in Ikenberry, ed., *American Foreign Policy*, 268–290.
11. Jeffrey Haynes, *An Introduction to International Relations and Religion*, 2nd ed. (London: Routledge, 2013); Peter Mandaville, "Islam and International Relations in the Middle East: From *Umma* to Nation State," in Louise Fawcett, ed., *International Relations of the Middle East*, 3rd ed. (Oxford: Oxford University Press, 2013), 167–184; Carolyn M. Warner and Stephen G. Walker, "Thinking About the Role of Religion in Foreign Policy: A Framework for Analysis," *Foreign Policy Analysis*, vol. 7 (2011): 113–135.
12. Hudson, *Foreign Policy Analysis*, 186.
13. Masoud Kazemzadeh, "Teaching the Politics of Islamic Fundamentalism," *PS: Political Science and Politics*, vol. 31 (1998): 52–59.
14. Ahmad Nizar Hamzeh, *In the Path of Hizbullah* (Syracuse, NY: Syracuse University Press, 2004), 32–36.
15. Kenneth Katzman, *Iran's Foreign Policy* (Washington, DC: Congressional Research Service, August 24, 2016), 10–15.
16. Mansour Farhang, "*Taamaoli Bar Mantegh Siasat Khareji Jomhuri Islami Iran*" (Thoughts on the Logic of the Foreign Policy of the Islamic Republic of Iran), BBC, July 25, 2012, available at http://www.bbc.co.uk/blogs/persian/viewpoints/2012/07/post-230.html (accessed July 29, 2012); Mehran Kamrava, "Iranian National-Security Debates: Factionalism and Lost Opportunities," *Middle East Policy*, vol. 14 (2007): 84–100; Mehdi Khalaji, *Apocalyptic Politics: On the Rationality of Iranian Politics* (Washington, DC: Washington Institute for Middle East Policy, 2008); Abbas Maleki, *Decision Making in Iran's Foreign Policy: A Heuristic Approach* (Tehran, Iran: International Institute for Caspian Studies, 2002), available at http://www.caspianstudies.com/article/Decision%20Making%20in%20Iran-FinalDraft.pdf (accessed June 20, 2012); Ali Akbar Rafsanjani, "*Mosahebeh ba Ayatollah Hashemi Rafsanjani: Vakavi Roykardha dar Howzeh Siasat Khareji*" (Interview with Ayatollah Hashemi Rafsanjani: Analyzing Viewpoints on the Realm of Foreign Policy), *Rahbord*, vol. 27 (2003): 5–30; Mahmoud Sariolghalam, "*Ya Ma Eshtebah Mikonim Ya Donya*" (Either We Are Making Mistakes Or the World Is Making Mistake), *Tabnak*, June 6, 2012, available at http://www.tabnak.ir/fa/news/249471 (accessed July 18, 2012).
17. I owe this argument to Valerie Hudson's comment on an earlier version of this article.
18. Holsti, 16.
19. Rouholamin Saeedi, "*Enghelabiyn Farsoodeh Va Toteeh Jam Zahr*" (Dilapidated Revolutionaries and the Conspiracy of Chalice of Poison), *Kayhan*, December 8, 2012, available at http://www.kayhannews.ir/910918/8.htm#other601 (accessed December 10, 2012), my translation.
20. Kazemzadeh, "Ayatollah Khamenei's Foreign Policy."
21. Kamrava, "Iranian National-Security Debates"; and Maleki, *Decision Making*.
22. Hussein Bastani, "*Afsaneh va Vaghiyat Dar Mored 'Mard Posht Pardeh' Dowlat Ahmadinejad*" (Myth and Reality on the 'Man Behind the Scenes' of Ahmadinejad's Government), BBC, September 16, 2012, available at http://www.bbc.co.uk/persian/iran/2012/09/120916_l39_analysis_khamenei_mashaei_ahmadinejad.shtml

(accessed September 18, 2012); Kasra Naji, *Ahmadinejad: The Secret History of Iran's Radical Leader* (Berkeley, CA: University of California Press, 2008).

23. Masoud Kazemzadeh, "Hassan Rouhani's Election and its Consequences for American Foreign Policy," *American Foreign Policy Interests*, vol. 36 (2014): 127–137.
24. Arash Bahmani, "*Gamaneh-zani Dar Bareh Dowlat Rouhani: Hamrahan Cabineh 'Tadbir va Omid' Cheh Kesani Hastand*" (Guessing about Rouhani's Government: Who Will Be in the Cabinet of 'Wisdom and Hope'), *Rooz Online*, June 20, 2013, available at http://www.roozonline.com/persian/news/newsitem/archive/2013/june/20/article/-fcf86e7d61.html (accessed June 21, 2013); BBC Persian, "*Rouhani Goruhi Ra 'Masoul Barasi Abad Mozakereh Bah Gorouh 5+1 Kardeh Ast'*" (Rouhani Has Chosen a Group 'For Assessing Various Dimension of the Negotiations with the Group of P5+1'), BBC, June 26, 2013, available at http://www.bbc.co.uk/persian/iran/2013/06/130626_mgh_iran_rouhani_nuclear.shtml (accessed June 27, 2013); Iran Emrooz, "*Mokhalefat Khamenei Ba Entekhab Yunesi Beh Onvan Vazir Ettelaat*" (Khamenei's Opposition to the Selection of Yunesi for the Position of Minister of Intelligence), June 28, 2013, available at http://www.iran-emrooz.net/index.php/news2/46360/ (accessed June 29, 2013).
25. Bahmani, ibid.
26. Maleki, *Decision Making*.
27. Bahmani, "*Gamaneh-zani*"; BBC Persian, "*Rouhani*"; and Iran Emrooz, "*Mokhalefat*."
28. Rafsanjani, "Mosahebeh ba Ayatollah Hashemi Rafsanjani."
29. Kamrava, "Iranian National-Security Debates."
30. Rafsanjani, "*Mosahebeh ba Ayatollah Hashemi Rafsanjani*"; Rafsanjani, "*Mosahebeh Ba Arman*" (Interview with Arman Newspaper), October 7, 2012, available at http://www.hashemirafsanjani.ir/fa/print/206158 (accessed October 7, 2012).
31. Hassan Rouhani, "*Mosahebeh*" (Interview), *Baztab*, July 22, 2006, available at http://www.baztab.ir/news/43515.php (accessed July 24, 2006).
32. Masoud Kazemzadeh, "Ahmadinejad's Foreign Policy," *Comparative Studies of South Asia, Africa and the Middle East*, vol. 27 (2007): 423–449; Masoud Kazemzadeh, "Intra-Elite Factionalism and the 2004 Majles Elections in Iran," *Middle Eastern Studies*, vol. 44 (2008): 189–214.
33. Masoud Kazemzadeh, "Ayatollah Khamenei's Foreign Policy Orientation," *Comparative Strategy*, vol. 32 (2013): 443–458.
34. Kazemzadeh, "Intra-Elite Factionalism."
35. Mohsen M. Milani, "Iran's Active Neutrality During the Kuwaiti Crisis: Reasons and Ramifications," *New Political Science*, vols. 21–22 (1992): 41–60.
36. Mohsen Aminzadeh, "*Kalbod-Shekafi 8 Sal Siasat Khareji Khatami*" (Dissection of the Eight Years of Khatami's Foreign Policy), Interview with Zhila Bani Yaaghub, part 1, *Gooya*, August 10, 2005, available at http://news.gooya.com/columnists/archives/034506.php (accessed July 28, 2012); Aminzadeh, "*Kalbod-Shekafi 8 Sal Siasat Khareji Khatami*" (Dissection of the Eight Years of Khatami's Foreign Policy), Interview with Zhila Bani Yaaghub, part 2, *Gooya*, August 10, 2005, available at http://news.gooya.com/columnists/archives/034507.php (accessed July 28, 2012); Aminzadeh, "*Siasat Hastehee Iran Va Peyamadhay Aan*" (Iran's Nuclear Policy and Its Consequences), *Gooya*, March 7, 2006, available at http://mag.gooya.com/politics/archives/2006/03/045138print.php (accessed July 28, 2012); Aminzadeh, "*Siasat Khareji Iran, Enteghal Az Charchoob Fekri Eslahat Beh Rahyaft Mohajem Va Tondro*" (Iran's Foreign Policy, Transition from the Framework of Reformist Thought to Offensive/Aggressive and Extremist Policy), *Gooya*, April 2, 2006, available at http://mag.gooya.com/politics/archives/2006/04/046129print.php (accessed July 28, 2012); Fatemeh Haghighatjoo, "Factional Positions on the Nuclear Issue in the Context of Iranian Domestic Politics," *Iran Analysis Quarterly*, vol. 3 (2006): 2–10; and Mohammad Reza Khatami, "Interview," *ILNA*, 2006, available at http://www.ilna.ir/print.asp?code=306058 (accessed September 15, 2007).
37. Jalil Roshandel, "Iran's Foreign and Security Policies: How the Decisionmaking Process Evolved," *Security Dialogue*, vol. 31 (200): 105–117.
38. Kaveh Afrasiabi and Abbas Maleki, "Iran's Foreign Policy After 11 September," *Brown Journal of World Affairs*, vol. 9 (2003): 255–265; Kamrava, "Iranian National-Security Debates"; Kazemzadeh, "Ahmadinejad's Foreign Policy"; Ali Khamenei, "Supreme Leader's Speech to Government Officials," July 24, 2012, available at http://english.khamenei.ir//index.php?option=com_content&task=view&id=1655&Itemid=4 (accessed July 29, 2012); and YouTube, "*Monazereh Shariatmadari va Asgharzadeh*" (Debate between Shariatmadari and Asgharzadeh), November 2, 2012, available at http://www.youtube.com/watch?v=-vd0oWeZT94& (accessed November 4, 2012).
39. Mehdi Perpinchi, "*Cheragh Sabz Eslah-talabha Dar Vaziyat Ghermez Hastehee*" (Green Light of the Reformists Under the Red Nuclear Condition), BBC, July 18, 2012, available at http://www.bbc.co.uk/persian/iran/2012/07/120718_ll_iran_politics.shtml (accessed July 19, 2012).
40. Perpinchi, ibid.; Rouholamin Saeedi, "*Enghelabiyn Farsoodeh.*
41. YouTube, Debate between Shariatmadari and Asgharzadeh.
42. Gary Samore, *The Iran Nuclear Deal: A Definitive Guide* (Cambridge, MA: Harvard University, 2015), available at http://belfercenter.ksg.harvard.edu/publication/25599/iran_nuclear_deal.html?breadcrumb=%2Fproject%2F77%2Firan_project (accessed March 27, 2016).

43. Ali Khamenei, "*Bayanat Dar Didar Asatid Daneshgah*" (Remarks in the Meeting with University Professors), August 30, 2009, available at http://farsi.khamenei.ir/speech-content?id=7959 (accessed September 10, 2009); YouTube, (Debate between Shariatmadari and Asgharzadeh).
44. Kamrava, "Iranian National-Security Debates"; Kazemzadeh, "Ahmadinejad's Foreign Policy"; Khalaji, *Apocalyptic Politics*; Khamenei, "Supreme Leader's Speech"; Karim Sadjadpour, *Reading Khamenei: The World View of Iran's Most Powerful Leader*, (Washington, DC: Carnegie Endowment for International Peace, 2008); Saeedi, "*Enghelabiyn*."
45. Golnaz Esfandiari, "Zionists Waiting to Kill Hidden Imam, Says Iranian Cleric," *Radio Free Europe/Radio Liberty*, September 1, 2010, available at http://www.rferl.org/content/Zionists_Waiting_To_Kill_Hidden_Imam_Says_Iranian_Cleric/2145806.html (accessed November 10, 2010); Khalaji, *Apocalyptic Politics*; Tabnak, "*Ahmadinejad: Sanad Darim America Mikhahad Joloyeh Zohour Imam Zaman Ra Begirad*" (Ahmadinejad: We Have Document on the U.S. Wanting to Prevent the Appearance of the 12th Imam), December 4, 2009, available at http://www.tabnak.ir/fa/pages/?cid=75711 (accessed December 5, 2010); YouTube, "CIA and MI6 Torture to Get Information on the Hidden Imam Zamaan In Iraq," program produced by the Iranian state television, March 18, 2011, available at http://www.youtube.com/watch?v=mkWT0fcSfg8 (accessed March 20, 2011).
46. ISNA, "*Saeedi: Sepah Yaki Az Abzarhay Zamineh Saz Zohor Imam Zaman (Aj) Ast*" (Saeedi: The IRGC is One of the Instruments for the Creation of Conditions for the Appearance of the 12th Imam), July 27, 2012, available at http://isna.ir/fa/news/91050603505 (accessed July 27, 2012).
47. Mahmoud Ahmadinejad, "U.S. Worried About Emam Zaman," Iranian, 2008, available at http://www.iranian.com/main/singlepage/2008/u-s-worried-about-emam-zaman (accessed June 1, 2008); Kazemzadeh, "Ahmadinejad's Foreign Policy"; Khalaji, *Apocalyptic Politics*.
48. BBC, "Iran Press Divided Over Geneva Deal," January 20, 2014, available at http://www.bbc.com/news/world-middle-east-25809977 (accessed November 30, 2014).
49. For an excellent study, see Kevjn Lim, "National Security Decision-Making in Iran," *Comparative Strategy*, vol. 34 (2015): 149–168. Also see Shahram Chubin, "The Politics of Iran's Nuclear Program," *The Iran Primer* (Washington, DC: U.S. Institute of Peace, 2010) available at https://www.wilsoncenter.org/sites/default/files/The%20Politics%20of%20Iran%2527s%20Nuclear%20Program.pdf (accessed September 25, 2016).
50. Michael R. Gordon, "Iran's Master of Iraq Chaos Still Vexes U.S.," *The New York Times*, October 2 2012.
51. Shahram Chubin, "Command and Control in a Nuclear-Armed Iran," *Proliferation Papers*, no. 45 (January–February 2013): 24.
52. "*Sardar Soleymani: Tahrimha Daha Barabar Ham Shavad, Iran Hemayatash Az Felestin Ra Ghat'a Nemikonad*" (Gen. Soleymani: Even if the Sanctions Are Multiplied by Factors of Tens, Iran Will Not Stop Its Support for Palestine), *Fars News*, March 17, 2016, available at http://www.farsnews.com/13941227000240 (accessed March 28, 2016).
53. Thomas Erdbrink, "Iran Tests More Missiles in Message to Israel and Biden," *The New York Times*, March 9, 2016.
54. AFP, "Iran Reveals Huge Underground Missile Base with Broadcast on State TV," *The Guardian*, October 15, 2015.
55. Jamie Crawford, "Close Encounter between U.S. Warship and Iranian Rocket," CNN, January 9, 2016, available at http://www.cnn.com/2015/12/29/politics/iran-missile-test-uss-harry-truman-aircraft-carrier/ (accessed April 6, 2016).
56. David Larter, "U.S. Navy Rebukes Iran after Propaganda Video Shows Sailor Crying," *Navy Times*, February 10, 2016, available at http://www.navytimes.com/story/military/2016/02/10/iran-images-riverine-crying-strong-condemnation-navy/80186322/ (accessed April 6, 2016).
57. Dan Lamothe, "Iranian Weapons Keep Getting Smuggled at Sea: Stopping Them Isn't Easy for the Navy," *The Washington Post*, April 5, 2016.
58. Rick Gladstone, "Iran Executions at Highest Level Since '89," *The New York Times*, March 10, 2016.
59. Ray Takeyh, "Introduction: What Do We Know?" in Robert D. Blackwill, ed., *Iran: The Nuclear Challenge* (New York: Council on Foreign Relations, 2012), 1.
60. Chubin, "The Politics of Iran's Nuclear Program."
61. IAEA, Report by the Director General, Implementation of the NPT Safeguards Agreement and relevant provisions of Security Council resolutions in the Islamic Republic of Iran, November 8, 2011, available at http://www.iaea.org/Publications/Documents/Board/2011/gov2011-65.pdf (accessed December 20, 2011), 8.
62. Takeyh, "Introduction," 2.
63. Haghighatjoo, "Factional Positions," 4, 8.
64. R. Jeffrey Smith and Joby Warrick, "Pakistan Scientist Khan Describes Iranian Efforts to Buy Nuclear Bombs," *The Washington Post*, March 14, 2010.
65. Kazemzadeh, "Hassan Rouhani's Election."
66. IAEA, Report by the Director General, Annex 1.
67. IAEA, ibid.
68. Aminzadeh, "Dissection"; Aminzadeh, "Iran's Foreign Policy"; Islamic Iran Participation Front, No Title, March 19, 2006 (published under the title "The Statement that Was Published After Six Years," October 21, 2012, available at http://www.iran-emrooz.net/index.php/news1/41410/ (accessed October 23, 2012); Haghighatjoo, "Factional Positions," 3.
69. Aminzadeh, "Iran's Nuclear Policy."

70. Ibid.
71. Ibid.
72. Ibid.
73. Ahmad Jennati, "*Ahmad Jennati: Masir Parvandeh Hastehi dar Do Sale Gozashte Na-dorost Bood*" (Ahmad Jennati: The Policy Trend of the Nuclear File in the Past Two Years Was Unsound), *ILNA*, February 17, 2006, available at http://www.ilna.ir/shownews.asp?code=281793&code1=1 (accessed February 20, 2006).
74. Khamenei, "Supreme Leader's Speech."
75. Islamic Iran Participation Front, "The Statement."
76. Ibid., my translation.
77. Ali Khamenei, "Supreme Leader's Letter to President Rouhani Regarding the Bar-Jaam," Khamenei.ir, October 21, 2015, available at http://english.khamenei.ir//index.php?option=com_content&task=view&id=2130 (accessed October 31, 2015).
78. Masoud Kazemzadeh, "Post-Khamenei Iran and American National Interests," *The Hill*, July 11, 2016.

Ayatollah Khamenei's Foreign Policy Orientation

MASOUD KAZEMZADEH

This article analyzes the beliefs and patterns of behavior of Iran's Supreme Leader Ayatollah Ali Khamenei in regards to the nature of politics, political conflicts, and the role of agency in shaping events, strategy, and tactics. To do so, it discusses Khamenei's personal background, ideological formation, personality, and foreign policy statements.

Introduction

Many scholars have argued that studying the background, psychology, ideology, speeches, and interviews of leaders could detect patterns of behavior.[1] James Barber, for example, came up with four personality types to help predict the performance of American presidents.[2] Byman and Pollack have argued that the aggressive and bellicose foreign policy of Iraq under Saddam Hussein and the cautious foreign policy of Syria under Hafez al-Assad, where the two countries had very similar regimes and polities, could be explained by the personalities of the two leaders.[3] Margaret Hermann developed the concept of Leadership Trait Analysis to assess and compare the patterns of decision making by leaders across large numbers.[4] In Alexander George's concept of Operational Code includes the beliefs of leaders on the nature of politics, political conflicts, the extent to which one could shape political outcomes, strategy, and tactics that could shape foreign policy decisions of leaders.[5]

In this article, relying upon a qualitative approach, I discuss personal and social background, ideological beliefs, personality, and foreign policy statements of Ayatollah Khamenei. Special attention is made to probe his beliefs on the nature of politics, political conflicts, and the role of agency, strategy, and tactics, as well as patterns of behavior.

Personal Background

There are very few studies and biographies of Seyyed Ali Husseni Khamenei.[6] Part of this has to do with his personality. Although very powerful, he has operated behind the scenes until the recent period. His own excellent website, which includes his biography and speeches, provides a venue to analyze him.

Khamenei was born on July 16, 1939, in the shrine city of Mashhad to a cleric of Azerbaijani background. His father, Seyyed Javad Husseni Khamanei, was a low-ranking cleric who operated a small mosque close to the shrine of the 8th Imam. The mosque catered primarily to the Azerbaijani population in Mashhad. The family lived in a one-room house with a basement. Later two rooms were added to the house. The family was not wealthy because Khamenei's father did not speak Persian well and was not an accomplished cleric, and the Azerbaijani population in Mashhad was very small. After his first wife died,

Javad Khamenei married a second wife, Ali Khamenei's mother. Ali Khamenei's mother, named Khadijeh, is a daughter of Ayatollah Hashem Mirdamadi, a cleric from Esfehan, who lived in Mashhad. Khamenei's father passed away at the age of 92 in 1986. His mother passed away in 1989, about two months after Khamenei became Supreme Leader in June 1989.[7]

Khamenei has three brothers and one sister, as well as three half-sisters from his father's first marriage. Khamenei is the second son in the family. All his brothers have had top government positions in the Islamic Republic of Iran (IRI). His older brother Mohammad and his younger brother Hadi are clerics as well. His youngest brother Hassan is the only male child who did not become a cleric. His brother Hadi is a reformist member of the fundamentalist oligarchy. His full sister, Badri, is married to Sheikh Ali Tehrani. Tehrani was one of the very top clerics in Mashhad and regarded as one of Ayatollah Ruhollah Khomeini's top students.[8]

Khamenei's father sent him to *maktab khaneh*, a theological primary school owned and taught by clerics. At the age of 12, he attended Soleyman Khan School, which was part of the seminary in Mashhad.[9] The students at Soleyman Khan were called *talabeh* (seminary student), and not *daneshamooz* (student, pupil). After Soleyman Khan, he went to the adult seminary and became a cleric. Khamenei did not attend a university.

Khamenei married Ms. Khojasteh in 1964. He was 25 years old and she was 17, which was very typical for religious families at that time. She was born into a very traditional religious family in Mashhad and had only a few years of education at a religious school for females run by a religious woman. In a 1992 interview with a fundamentalist women's magazine, Mrs. Khojasteh-Khamenei says: "I married him in 1964. Of course this marriage took place before we became acquainted with each other, since as was the practice of religious families of those days, his mother came to our house to propose and after the usual discussions the marriage ceremonies were performed."[10] They have four sons (from the oldest to the youngest, Mostafa, Mojtaba, Mohsen Masoud, and Meysam) and two daughters (from older to younger, Bashri and Hoda). The sons were born before the revolution and the daughters were born after the revolution. The first three sons (Mostafa, Mojtaba, and Mohsen Masoud) are clerics. The two daughters have high-school degrees from Refah High School, a private school with very heavy religious content whose students come from very religious families both before and after the revolution.[11]

Mostafa is married to the daughter of Ayatollah Azizollah Khoshvaght. Khoshvaght (died February 2013) was one of the most right-wing hard-line clerics in the oligarchy. Khoshvaght was very close to Ayatollah Mesbah Yazdi, who is the most extreme hard-line leader among the top echelon of the oligarchy. Mojtaba is married to the daughter of Gholam-Ali Haddad-Adel. Haddad-Adel, a conservative hard-liner, was a professor of Islamic philosophy and Speaker of the Majlis. Haddad-Adel is currently a member of *the* Majlis and senior adviser to Khamenei. Mohsen Masoud is married to the daughter of Ayatollah Kharrazi. Bashri is married to the son of Ayatollah Mohammad Mohammadi Golpaygani, who is Khamenei's chief of staff.[12]

The eldest son, Mostafa, went to the war front and participated in the war with Iraq. The second son, Mojtaba, was born in the Iranian calendar year 1348 H.S. (March 20, 1969–March 20, 1970). After he finished high school in 1366 H.S. (1987 A.D.), at the age of 18, Mojtaba went to the war front and participated in the war against Iraq. The years 1987–88 were among the bloodiest years of the war when Saddam was using chemical weapons on Iranian troops. At the time, Khamenei was the president of Iran. It is significant to note that not only did Khamenei spend time at the war front, but he also sent his sons who were old enough to participate in the war to the war front.[13]

Ideological Beliefs

Khamenei has been a fundamentalist since he was 13 years old. He was introduced to fundamentalism while attending the Solayman Khan School, when he first heard Navab Safavi speak at his school in 1952. Khamenei says that he was greatly influenced by Navab Safavi when he heard him talk at his school and the following day at the Navab Madrasah seminary.[14] In his biography on his website, Khamenei writes:

> . . . The very first sparks of consciousness concerning Islamic, revolutionary ideas and the duty to fight the Shah's despotism and his British supporters, was kindled in my soul at the age of 13 when the brave cleric, Nawwab Safavi, later martyred by the Shah's regime, came to our school in Mashhad in 1952 and delivered a fiery speech against the Shah's anti-Islamic and devious policies.[15]

Before the 1979 revolution, there were four groups that may be classified as fundamentalist or pre-fundamentalist. The first fundamentalist organization in Iran is the Fadaian Islam (Self-Sarificers of Islam). The Fadaian Islam has been the most extreme and the most violent fundamentalist group in Iran. The Fadaian Islam was founded by Navab Safavi in 1945.[16] Safavi was inspired by the Muslim Brotherhood in Egypt. Unlike the Egyptian Brotherhood, the Fadaian Islam was primarily a terrorist organization. The Fadaian Islam assassinated Ahmad Kasravi on March 11, 1946, and Prime Minister Gen. Ali Razmara on March 7, 1951. Kasravi was one of Iran's most prominent historians and secular intellectuals. Razmara, an independent, was prime minister at the time. The Fadaian Islam also made unsuccessful assassination attempts on Dr. Hussein Fatemi on February 16, 1952, Abdul-Hussein Hazhir on November 4, 1949, and Hussein Ala on November 17, 1955. Fatemi, a liberal democrat, was Mossadegh's foreign minister and number-two leader of the pro-democracy Iran National Front. Hazhir, a monarchist, was court minister and former prime minister. Hussein Ala, a monarchist, was prime minister. The Fadaian Islam also had a plan to assassinate Dr. Mossadegh, a liberal democrat, when he was prime minister.[17]

The Fadaian Islam advocated an Islamic government, implementation of Shariah, banning the sale and consumption of alcohol, imposition of compulsory hijab on women, and gender segregation of all schools, among others. Its leader after the revolution was Ayatollah Sadegh Khalkhali, known as the "hanging judge" after the revolution for his summary executions of monarchists, Marxists, and ethnic minority activists. Khalkhali was a long-time friend of Ayatollah Ruhollah Khomeini from the days that they were young clerics. Mohammad Mehdi Abd-Khodae, Fatemi's would-be assassin, is the current secretary-general and number-one leader of the Fadaian Islam.[18] Abd-Khodae is a hard-line fundamentalist and was a member of the Majlis after the revolution.

The second fundamentalist group is the Hezb Motalefeh Islami (Islamic Coalition Party). Still active, the party is anchored among the traditional bazaars and advocates traditional conservative social mores as well as non-statist economic policies. Their policies have remained remarkably consistent since the revolution. Most of their leaders have become extremely wealthy bazaar merchants after the revolution.

A third group that is not fundamentalist, but from which many fundamentalist leaders emerged, is the Hojatieh Society. "Hojat" is one of the names of the 12th Imam. The Hojatieh Society was related to those who were waiting for the reappearance of the 12th Imam, the Shia Islam's Messiah. It was a right-wing group that was strongly anticommunist. It also promoted bigoted views against the Bahais. It had a very close working relationship with SAVAK, the Shah's secret police. Hojatieh was against the notion that one should struggle against the Shah. It was also against the notion that it was either possible or desirable to have an Islamist government. It believed in the notion that one should wait for the reappearance of the 12th Imam.

Although the Hojatieh Society as an organization did not participate in the revolution during 1978 to 1979, many of its members left it and joined Khomeini between 1978 and 1984. Many top officials of the IRI were members of the Hojatieh. Because it was a semi-secret society, many of its members deny that they have been members. After the revolution, Khomeini condemned the group but welcomed its former members into high ranks of the new oligarchy. Some of the top members of the Hojatieh who became part of the fundamentalist oligarchy are Ali Akbar Velayati, Parvaresh, and Abdolkarim Soroush.[19] Velayati served as the powerful foreign minister between 1981 and 1997. Since 1997, Velayati has been the senior foreign policy adviser to the supreme leader. Parvaresh served as the minister of education in the 1980s. Soroush was one of the architects of the Cultural Revolution—which purged the universities from liberal, secular, Marxist, and leftist professors, administrators, and students—and a one of the main thinkers among fundamentalists in the 1980s. Soroush was among one of the earliest members of the oligarchy who became a reformist.

The fourth group constitutes Khomeini and his supporters from 1963 onward. Khomeini began his political and religious activities from the early 1940s. In his first booklet, *Kashef al Asrar* (1943), Khomeini was openly and explicitly monarchist and a traditional Shia.[20] Khomeini was an assistant to Grand Ayatollah Brujerdi, the highest ranking cleric in Iran at the time and a monarchist. After the 1953 coup, Khomeini took secret messages from Brujerdi to the Shah.[21] Khomeini remained a monarchist until 1963. The reforms in June 1963 on land reform, female franchise, and changing the oath from the Quran to a holy book (which would have allowed Christians, Jews, Bahais, and Zoroastrians to hold high office) made Khomeini oppose the Shah and soon the system of monarchy. Khomeini gradually evolved from an ultra-conservative to a fundamentalist, with many reversals in his public political pronouncements.[22]

Soon after the overthrow of the Shah, the fundamentalists established the Islamic Republican Party (IRP) as the main fundamentalist party in Iran. Khamenei was one of the founders of the IRP. The primary goal of the IRP was to get rid of the secular democrats of the Iran National Front (who constituted about a third of the Provisional Government's cabinet), liberal Islamist Mehdi Bazargan (who was the prime minister in the Provisional Government), liberal Islamist AbolHassan Bani Sadr (elected president in January 1980 with about 75 percent of the votes cast), Marxist Islamist group the People's Mojahedin Organization of Iran (PMOI, also known as MKO, MEK), and the socialist left, all of whom participated in the revolution. The IRP wanted to create an Islamist system based on the rule of the Shia clerics and the Shariah. By June 1981, the IRP and Khomeini succeeded in purging all the non-fundamentalists from positions of power and establishing their full control. Although extremist and violent, Khomeini always was very pragmatic.

Unlike Ayatollah Ruhollah Khomeini, Ali Khamanei has always been a fundamentalist. He was first attracted to Navab Safavi and the Fadaian Islam.[23] Khamenei translated two of Sayyid Qutb's books: *An Indictment against the Western Civilization,* and *The Future in Islamic Lands.* Qutb was the primary theoretician of the Muslim Brotherhood, whose writings constitute the pillar of all fundamentalists (Sunni and Shia alike, from the Egyptian Muslim Brotherhood to al Qaeda to Iran's Fadaian Islam). In 1963, when Khomeini began opposing the Shah, Khamenei (at age 24) joined the protests and began supporting Khomeini. This was the first political act by Khamenei.[24] While Khomeini was supporting the Shah and monarchy (i.e., before June 1963), Khamenei was not supporting Khomeini's pro-Shah policies. Khamenei had been supporting the Fadaian Islam. Khamenei has repeatedly and publicly supported the views of Navab Safavi.

Khamenei was not, and is not, an erudite theological scholar or thinker. None of his cohorts at the seminary school has mentioned that he was a particularly good student.[25] According to Grand Ayatollah Hussein Ali Montazeri, who was his teacher, Khamenei lacks the theological qualifications to issue a fatwa (religious decree).[26] His power is due to his political activities, support for Khomeini, and great oratorical skills. Moreover, between February 1979 and June 1989, many senior fundamentalist clerics were killed: they included Ayatollah Mohammad Beheshti, Ayatollah Morteza Motahhari, and Hojatolislam Mohammad Javad Bahonar. Several months before Khomeini died, his designated successor Grand Ayatollah Hussein Ali Montazeri was dismissed due to his opposition to mass executions of political prisoners as well as his opposition to the rape of virgin female political prisoners before their executions. Khamenei's selection to the position of supreme leader by the Assembly of Experts after Khomeini died in June 1989 was due to the determining role of Rafsanjani, who had been Khamenei's friend since around 1957. Rafsanjani was one of two clerics who were exceptionally close friends with Khomeini for many decades. The other cleric was Ayatollah Sadegh Khalkhali.[27]

Personality Character

Khamenei's personality contains some apparently contradictory features. On the one hand, he is a true believer, who has embraced and advocated extreme views and lives them. On the other hand, he hides some of his more extreme views only to be revealed after he has accomplished his goal.

Khamenei is a true believer. Between 1963 and 1978, Khamenei was sent to prison six times for his activities against the Shah and in support of Khomeini. He spent about three years in prison. He says that he was tortured by SAVAK.[28] He also lived clandestinely for about one year in 1345 H.S. (circa 1967 A.D.) in Tehran. He was sent to internal exile.[29] At Khamenei's official website under the section "Others' Memories" of Khamenei, there is a memory from the son of Seyyed Ali Andarzgoo (a militant cleric who engaged in armed struggle against the Shah before the revolution), which states that Andarzgoo held classes on how to use arms for several militants including Khamenei, martyred Hasheminejad, and Ayatollah Vaez Tabasi.[30] After the revolution, Khamenei survived an assassination attempt which permanently disabled his right hand.[31] While president, Khamenei visited the war front numerous times and spent time with the IRGC fighters at the front.[32] Moreover, he sent his sons, Mostafa and Mojtaba, to serve as fighters in the bloody Iran-Iraq war front.[33]

Another major personality characteristic of Khamenei has been his repeated hiding of his more extreme views and policies. The stealthy nature of Khamenei's real views and policy preferences has confused his supporters and rivals within the fundamentalist oligarchy and those outside it. Only much later has it become clear exactly what policies or persons were favored by Khamenei.

For example, Khamenei's acquiescence to the nuclear agreements with the EU3 (the UK, France, and Germany) and the International Atomic Energy Agency (IAEA) in 2003–2004 on accepting the Additional Protocols and suspension of uranium enrichment were understood as his support for these agreements. However, in 2012 he strongly condemned the reformists and expedients (Rafsanjani's faction) for having made those agreements. Only after Khamenei was able to sideline reformists and expedients and replace them with the hard-line Ahmadinejad and enact more extreme policies in regards to the nuclear program did Khamenei reveal his true policy.[34]

Another example is the treatment of Rafsanjani. By 2009, Khamenei and Rafsanjani had been close friends for about 52 years. He owed his position of being the supreme leader to Rafsanjani's determining role at the Assembly of Experts. Still, Khamenei was willing to have his proxies publicly humiliate Rafsanjani, strip him of much of his powers, and even have his daughter Faezeh and son Mehdi put in jail on political charges in September 2012.

What these examples indicate is that it has been extremely hard to decipher exactly what have been Khamenei's political objectives and policy preferences. Unlike other actors such as Rafsanjani or the reformists, who explicitly state their policies, Khamenei has had a long track record of hiding some of his preferences. It is, therefore, hard to know exactly what are some of Khamenei's real short-term and long-term objectives and preferences.

However, the historical record is strong on several personal characteristics of Khamenei. Khamenei has been a violent extremist fundamentalist all his adult life. He intensely hates and opposes the U.S. and Israel. He tends to camouflage his tactics and has been very good at them.[35] He has shown a great ability to deceive and surprise even his closest friends and allies, such as Rafsanjani. Khamenei tends to say one thing in public and do the opposite in action. For example, he condemns dictatorship and praises democracy, while he knows for certain that there is no democracy or freedom of expression in Iran.[36]

Therefore, not everything Khamenei says should be taken at face value. For example, Khamenei has issued a fatwa declaring nuclear weapons forbidden. However, a *fatwa* could easily be changed when circumstances change. Moreover, Shias are allowed *taghiyeh* (dissimulation, or lying) under some circumstances. Khamenei's predecessor, Khomeini, elevated the notion of *maslahat* (expediency, interests) as a primary value in the Islamic Republic. Therefore, it would be very easy for Khamenei to simply state in a second fatwa that it was *maslahat* (expedient) to deceive the enemies with the first fatwa in order to promote the interests of Islam or the Islamic Republic. After all, when in Paris, Khomeini promised that he would establish democracy, freedom (even for Marxists), that he would not take any position of power, and that clerics would not become presidents. But as soon as he was able to, Khomeini established a theocracy, made himself the supreme leader for life, mass executed Marxists, harshly repressed secular democrats, and even placed under house arrest and publicly humiliated on national television the highest ranking cleric in Iran, Grand Ayatollah Kazem Shariatmadari. The IAEA has documented actual evidence of Iran's nuclear weapons dimensions, including an indigenous nuclear weapons design.[37] The revelations documented by the IAEA are in stark contrast to Khamenei's repeated claims that Iran's nuclear programs have solely peaceful dimensions. The evidence has been so strong that even China and Russia, Iran's allies, have supported several resolutions against the Islamic Republic at the UN Security Council.

Khamenei is a believer in *estekhareh* (bibliomancy).[38] *Estekhareh* is used to decide what to do. In Iran, the Quran's pages are marked "good" or "bad." In *estekhareh*, after the recitation of a prayer, the person randomly opens a page of the Quran. If the page is marked "good" then the person goes ahead with the deal, and if the page is marked "bad" then the person does not make the deal.

Ideologue or Pragmatic?

Is Khamenei an ideologue or a realist/pragmatic when it comes to foreign and defense policies? Does he make decisions based on rational cost-benefit calculations or is he motivated by his fundamentalist ideology?

The debate in Iran is whether Iran's foreign policy is based on ideology (of Shia fundamentalism) or is it based on rational pragmatic cost-benefit analysis to protect and promote Iran's national interests. The division first began in early 1979. The provisional government (composed of secular democrats and liberal Islamists) wanted the personnel appointed to various offices to be competent and foreign policy decisions to be made to advance Iran's national interests based on rational cost-benefit analysis. Khomeini, and the IRP, instead wanted the personnel to be primarily ideologues and foreign policy to be based on the ideals of the revolution. The debate was called *Motekhases* (expert, specialist, competent) vs. *Maktabi* (ideologue, ideological).

Some of the ideological foreign policy goals of the fundamentalists have been: export of the revolution via undermining of various regimes in the Middle East and assisting their radical opponents; opposition to the current international system; opposition to the U.S.; opposition to the state of Israel and the two-state solution; and assistance to various radical Islamic fundamentalist groups such as Lebanese Hezbollah, Hamas, and Palestinian Islamic Jihad (PIJ). Since 1997, the reformist members of the oligarchy have called for the goals of Iran's foreign policy to be based on protecting and advancing the national interests of Iran instead of sacrificing the interests of Iran in pursuit of ideological goals. Reformists have argued that these ideological goals and policies harm the national interests by hurting the economy, undermining political stability of the regime, and possibly causing wars and costly confrontations with powerful global and regional actors.

When Rafsanjani was president (1989–1997), he wanted to hold negotiations with the U.S. Khamenei strongly opposed rapprochement and détente with the U.S.[39] According to Hussein Shariatmadari—who is one of the ideologues of the ultra hard-line faction, the representative of the supreme leader at the *Keyhan* daily, the editor-in-chief of *Keyhan*, and is extremely close to Khamenei—during Rafsanjani's presidency, Ataollah Mohajerani, the deputy to the president for legal affairs, advocated direct negotiations with the U.S.[40] Shariatmadari says that Khamenei argued that: "direct negotiations would ultimately lead to a deal, deal means give and take, the U.S. wants Iran to give up the pure Islam in the government and to stop the resistance (to the U.S. hegemony in the region and the world)."[41]

Central to Khamenei's foreign policy are his conceptions of the nature of the U.S. and the nature of the conflict between the Islamic Republic and the U.S. On December 6, 2012, Khamenei's website published a compilation of Khamenei's views on the nature of the conflict between the U.S. and the Islamic Republic in the form of answers to 10 questions based on his speeches since he became supreme leader.[42] One question was: "What is the primary reason for the enmity of the U.S. towards the people of Iran and the Islamic Republic?" In a speech on 24/09/1387 (December 14, 2008), Khamenei said:

> The reason for the deep and irreconcilable enmity of the Arrogance and its head the U.S. and the global Zionist network toward the Islamic Republic is . . . those things which the Islamic Republic opposes . . . Opposition to exploitation, opposition to domination, opposition to humiliation of the people by the world's political powers, opposition to political dependence, opposition to interference and penetration of dominant powers of the world, opposition to ethical secularism, opposition to libertines, these are things that the Islamic Republic absolutely opposes.[43]

Another question was: "What is the fundamental reason for us to confront the U.S. government?" In a speech delivered on 30/05/1385 (August 21, 2006), Khamenei said:

> Today the great idolatrous in the world is the regime of the United States of America; because Zionism created it and affirms it. America has replaced the former great idolatrous that was the British. ... Condemnation of the idolatrous is necessary.[44]

Another question was: "After this struggle what country has been the victor in the field?" In a speech delivered on 10/08/1391 (October 31, 2012), Khamenei said:

> When we understood that here the one who has become victorious is the people with decisive will and determination based on faith and dependence on god, then this becomes a lesson for all the peoples; this becomes a principle for all historical developments; a new philosophy of history based on Islamic principles, with observing this event [U.S.–Iran confrontation], develops, codifies, and then becomes accepted by all the others; and this is the reality which has occurred; meaning that the people of Iran all this time and until today has been the victor in this field... There is no one in the world who would doubt that in the past 30 years, the U.S. has declined more than 30 rankings in terms of power and global legitimacy; everybody sees this and knows this; the Americans themselves confess to this also.America has crashed. Today no government in the world is as despised as the government of America.[45]

The final question was: "What would be the end result of the historical struggle of the people of Iran with the arrogant government of America?" In a speech delivered on 28/05/1386 (August 19, 2007), Khamenei said:

> We are certain that in this fight between the righteous and the wrong that is going on today—the fight between Islam, Islamic teachings, and Islamic awakening on the one hand and the avaricious arrogant policies of the satans of the world and at their head, the Great Satan that is the government of America on the other hand—victory is with us; victory is with the side of the righteous. On this, there exists no doubt. All the evidence show and confirm this. The nature of god's traditions is also this; therefore, that other than this could have no meaning. The group that supports righteousness if they stand up and engage in action, there is no doubt that they will win against the wrong. God's traditions are on the side of strengthening the righteous and the natural expectation of the path of God's traditions in history also necessitates this. We are also, based on experience, observing this.[46]

Khamenei does not oppose talks with the U.S. as a matter of principle. He has allowed "topical talks" with the U.S. on issues such as Afghanistan, Iraq, or drug trafficking, or multilateral talks which include the U.S., such as those conducted under the aegis of the P5+1 (permanent members of the UN Security Council plus Germany) over the nuclear issue. However, his position on the sensitive notion of "comprehensive negotiations" with the U.S. to resolve the conflicts between the two countries has not been consistent. At some junctures, Khamenei has absolutely opposed such comprehensive negotiations due to what he considers to be the natures of the U.S. and Iran. But at other junctures, he has said that he might decide to have such negotiations under certain conditions.[47]

Since January 2009, the Obama administration, publicly and privately, has repeatedly offered bilateral direct negotiations to resolve the differences between the U.S. and Iran.

According to Khamenei, Obama in his confidential letters has stated that the policy of his administration is not regime change, that he respects him and the Iranian people, and that he wants direct bilateral negotiations to resolve the differences between the two countries.[48] Khamenei has refused to authorize direct bilateral comprehensive negotiations between his representatives and American officials. Khamenei emphasized that no representative from his office has ever negotiated with American officials. He added that officials from the government (i.e., the executive branch or the Supreme National Security Council) have been allowed to negotiate on topical issues and that they had to respect the leader's red lines, including bilateral talks with Americans at the sidelines of the P5+1 negotiations held in 2013.[49] Earlier, on February 16, 2013, in a major speech, Khamenei provided his reasons for rejecting Obama's offer of comprehensive negotiations. He said:

> First, . . . American officials are illogical people, their sayings are illogical, their actions are illogical, they are bullies, they expect others to surrender to their bullying and illogical actions. Well, some surrender . . . ,but the people of Iran and the system of the Islamic Republic is not the surrendering type . . . . When they say "We will not allow Iran to develop nuclear weapons," is a deception. Is the issue over nuclear weapons? On the issue of Iran's nuclear program, the issue is not over nuclear weapons; the issue is that you [the U.S.] want to prevent the definite and certain rights of the Iranian people to enrich uranium and the peaceful use of it based on its own domestic capabilities . . . The American officials say [these] illogical sayings. With illogical people, a person cannot sit and talk based on logic. Well, they are illogical, and illogical means they are bullies and say nonsense. This is the reality that we clearly learned in the past 30 years of confronting various global things. We know who is in front of us and how to deal with them . . . When they talk, when the president of the United States talks . . . [it] is to deceive the public opinion, the world public opinion, the public opinion of the peoples of the region, or if they could the public opinion of our own people.
>
> Second, . . . their intention is for propaganda to show to the Moslem peoples that see this system of the Islamic Republic with all its steadfastness and all its resistance, eventually was compelled to begin the process of negotiations and compromise. When the people of Iran has done this, what the rest of you [Muslim peoples] say? They [the Americans] need this in order to extinguish and demoralize the rising Moslem peoples who for dear Islam feel dignity and a breeze of awakening is blowing there. After the [1979] revolution, this was one of their goals. From the early years of the revolution, one of their goals was to bring Iran to the table for compromise and give-and-take. So that they could say, see eventually Iran that claimed that it was independent, standing up, fearless, and brave, was forced to come and sit at the negotiations table . . . Well, it is clear that the Islamic Republic is not naïve . . . ,it knows your goals; therefore, it gives you the response commensurate with your intentions.
>
> The third point is that negotiations in American practice and that of the dominating powers mean that come and sit and talk so that you accept our position . . . Lets come and sit so that we can convince Iran to stop enrichment, stop nuclear energy. This is the objective. They don't say, let's come, sit, and negotiate so that Iran can present its evidence, to stop the pressures over the nuclear issue, to stop the sanctions, to stop interfering in the security and political [affairs]. They say lets negotiate so that Iran would accept our sayings.

> The fourth point: in their propaganda they pretend that if Iran sits at the negotiating table with the U.S., the sanctions would be removed. This is another of their lies. Their goal is to use the promise of removing of sanctions so that they can compel the Iranian people to have enthusiasm for negotiations with the U.S . . . negotiations mean you accept our position, surrender, so that we would remove the sanctions. Well, if the people of Iran wanted to surrender, why did they do the revolution? . . . The people of Iran carried out the revolution so that they would get out of the yoke of America; now they come, sit and again surrender to you?
>
> The last point: Unlike them, we are logical . . . We accept logical sayings and logical actions. The Americans show that they are not bullies, show that they do not engage in wickedness, show that in their words and actions they do not say and do illogical things. Show that they respect the rights of the people of Iran, show that they do not enflame the region, show that they do not interfere in the affairs of Iran, like when they interfered during the July 2009 conspiracy, and supported the rioters . . . They do not do these things, then they can see that the system of the Islamic Republic is a system with good intentions. The path toward interaction with the Islamic Republic is only what we said and nothing else; on this path they could have interaction with the Islamic Republic. The Americans have to prove their good intentions.[50]

Basically, Khamenei regards the U.S. to be a "bullying" force which leads the *estekbar jahani* (global arrogance or global oppression), determined to dominate the world and undermine Islamic government, values, and power. By *estekbar jahani*, Khamenei means the international system under American control, which has come to be based on capitalism, liberal democracy, and secularism. Khamenei regards his role to be the leader of all the Muslims and Iran's role to be the leader of the "resistance bloc." The resistance bloc includes countries and movements that resist the current international system and includes Iran, Assad's regime in Syria, Lebanese Hezbollah, Hamas, and the PIJ. Khamenei believes that the U.S. and the West are in decline and that Iran and the Islamist groups are on the rise. Khamenei believes that the U.S. is too weak to impose its will on Iran.

Khamenei has been pursuing a policy of stalling and buying time. Exactly for what purpose Khamenei is stalling is not clear. Khamenei may be buying time until Iran completes its nuclear weapons program,[51] or until the U.S. collapses (similar to the collapse of communism and the USSR), or until the Americans leave the Middle East due to military and financial problems. In the meantime, Khamenei has been pursuing policies such as gradually developing Iran's nuclear program, bleeding Americans via proxies (e.g., Hezbollah, Muqtada al-Sadr's Jeish al-Mahdi) in the region, and attacking Israel via Hezbollah, Hamas, and PIJ.

Several pragmatic hard-liners (e.g., Tehran mayor and IRGC Gen. Mohammad Baqer Qalibaf, former Supreme Commander of the IRGC Gen. Mohsen Rezaee, and Head of the Majlis Ali Larijani) have publicly expressed worries and have blamed Ahmadinejad for unnecessarily endangering Iran by his bellicose policies.[52] However, at least since 2009, Ahmadinejad has repeatedly and publicly advocated negotiations with the U.S. And since 2010, it has been Khamenei who publicly has increasingly taken the most bellicose positions among the top members of the oligarchy. By mid-2012, many members of the oligarchy have expressed their serious concerns about pursuing an ideological foreign policy if that would result in an American invasion and regime change in Iran.

On July 24, 2012, Khamenei presented a major speech to the top government officials articulating his foreign policy doctrine.[53] The purpose of Khamenei's address was to undermine the arguments by the reformists and supporters of Rafsanjani, to respond to hard-liners who were worried, and to reassure his core hard-line base.

Khamenei agrees with the distinction between *arman-garayee* (idealism, ideology-driven) and *vaghebini* (realism, pragmatism, realistic). Khamenei wants to articulate a combination of idealism and realism. For Khamenei, both goals and means are determined by the combination of idealism and realism.

A close analysis of Khamenei's speech, however, shows that instead of combining idealism (or ideology) and realism (pragmatic analysis), he confuses the two during much of his speech. Khamenei argues that it is pragmatic-realistic to pursue the ideals/ideology of the Islamic revolution. He argues that wise methods could help achieve the ideals of the IRI. Khamenei wants to articulate that the IRI can use war against the U.S. and win and spread the power and ideals of the IRI.

From February 1979, Khomeini and Islamic fundamentalists have opposed the U.S. and called for the overthrow of various regimes in the region such as those in Iraq, Saudi Arabia, Jordan, and Egypt. The reactions of the governments in the region and the U.S. to the IRI's foreign policy have been to counter the IRI. Khamenei's refusal to change such policies and instead calling them a reaction to the West's hostility to the nature of the IRI does not make these ideological policies pragmatic-realist. Khamenei's primary goals remain the ideological objectives of opposing and defeating the current international system, the U.S., Israel, and various regimes in the region.

When it comes to the means, Khamenei wants to use a realist approach to observe the powers of Iran and its opponents. In this regard, although Khamenei's approach is realistic, his actual analysis is badly flawed, as the text of Khamenei's speech clearly shows. For example, Khamenei says that Iran is stronger than the combination of the U.S., Israel, and the EU. Khamenei argues that the U.S., Israel, and the EU are far weaker today than they were in the 1980s, while the IRI is far more powerful in 2012 than it was in the 1980s. For Khamenei, if they (U.S., Israel, and Western Europe) could not defeat Iran in the Iran–Iraq war (1980–1988), they could not defeat Iran today. Khamenei says (in this speech as well as in other speeches) that the war between Iran and the U.S. will be like the battles of Badr (624 A.D.) and Khaybar (629 A.D.), two seventh-century battles in which much smaller Islamic armies defeated enemies who possessed greater resources. Khamenei says the true supporters of the IRI should be willing to pay the costs and sacrifices of the war, and that eventually the IRI will win.

There is no mention of the 12th Imam's reappearance due to this war in this speech or in any other speech by Khamenei. What is interesting is that although many top officials appointed by Khamenei have publicly stated that we live at the age of the reappearance of the 12th Imam, Khamenei himself has neither articulated such viewpoints nor criticized them.[54] As of this writing, he has not revealed his own viewpoint on this subject, but has allowed others to articulate and spread messianic and apocalyptic viewpoints. Khamenei regularly visits the Jamkaran Mosque in Qom, where many believe that the 12th Imam hides in the well there.[55]

Although Khamenei says that he believes that Iran will win in a war against the U.S., Europe, and Israel, he nevertheless is also willing to engage in a war in which Iran would lose and he would die. In response to other fundamentalists who have been pressuring Khamenei to back down to pressure from the U.S., Khamenei has said: "If the enemy puts a lot of pressure here, what happened in Karbala will happen here."[56]

Karbala refers to the Battle of Karbala, where the Third Shia Imam, Hussein, was killed in a war against the forces of Yazid, the Sunni ruler. Shias celebrate martyrdom, including mass martyrdom as committed by the Third Shia Imam, Hussein, when he and 72 of his followers died in a mass suicide operation in Karbala against a formidable Sunni force on October 10, 680 A.D. Ashura refers to commemoration of the anniversary of the rebellion, defeat, and killing of the Third Shia Imam, Hussein, and his supporters (which included his children and other family members) by Yazid's army. The confrontation occurred during October 1–10, 680 A.D. in Karbala, in present-day Iraq. The Shias believe this episode teaches that Imam Hussein consciously decided to engage in mass martyrdom in order to preserve the Shia religion. At Karbala, Imam Hussein sacrificed not only his own life, but also the lives of his own sons Ali Akbar and Ali Asghar. Ashura thus teaches the necessity of martyrdom, including mass suicidal martyrdom. Every year during the first ten days of the Islamic month of Muharram, the Shia engage in numerous activities such as processions, ritual passion plays, sermons, and self-flagellations. Ashura events are thus powerful socialization events for the Shia faithful. The Shia fundamentalists have transformed the Karbala story into a powerful pillar of their ideology.

Khamenei explains his views on the lessons of Karbala in a sermon on Friday, October 18, 1983:

> On the day of Ashura, after his companions with both tears and insistence asked for permission and entered the battlefield and fought and were martyred, and nobody other than the youth of the Bani Hashem remained—the group devoted to Hoseyn Ebn-e Ali(AS)—Ali Akbar was the first youth to approach Imam Hoseyn (AS) and asked for permission to enter the battlefield. He came to Imam Hoseyn, who—and here is the remarkable thing—Imam Hoseyn, without the slightest hesitation, gave Ali Akbar permission to go to the battlefield . . .
>
> He went to the battlefield and fought until he was exhausted, and being a brave youth he was able to fight his way through the ranks of the enemy and return to his father. He said to Imam Hoseyn (AS) "O father, I am dying of thirst." Clearly there was no water in the camp of Imam Hoseyn Ebn-e Ali (AS). Therefore, he said "My son, go and continue fighting in the path of God! Soon you will be drinking from the hand of the Prophet (SAS)." Shortly thereafter everyone heard Ali Akbar's voice from the middle of the battlefield saying "Father, peace be unto you." "Goodbye my father." "This is my grandfather the Prophet of God."
>
> . . . Brothers and sisters [who have gathered here for prayers]! Make pious faith in God your calling, as you follow [the example of] Hoseyn Ebn-e Ali (AS), and his companions, and his youthful supporters, and his children. "O Creator! Cause us to be among his companions and supporters." (Amen from those congregated for prayers). "O Creator! Cause us to be among the people of Karbala."[57]

Conclusion

Khamenei's personal and social backgrounds are from a very traditional premodern clerical family. At a very early age, he embraced the violent extremist path of Navab Safavi. All his adult life, Khamenei has been an extremist fundamentalist. He is a true believer who has openly advocated extreme views and has paid greatly in personal costs. At the same time, he is very patient and is able to hide his most extreme views and policies until he can accomplish his goals. This does not means that he is realist/pragmatic in the sense that objectives and means are calculated based on cost-benefit analysis. Rather, the objectives and means could be very irrational, or even lead to mass suicidal deaths such as a war with the U.S. (along with Israel and the West). Khamenei's foreign policy goals are ideological, such as opposing the current international system as well as confronting the U.S. and Israel. And his willingness in the confrontation with the U.S. to pursue means along the model of Karbala—that is, a mass suicidal war against a much more powerful opponent—does not conform to a rational cost-benefit analysis. However, both these goals and means are consistent with the fundamentalist Shia ideology. The pragmatism in Khamenei is his willingness and ability to hide and dissimulate his policies and views until later when he could accomplish his ideologically derived goals and methods.

In sum, Khamenei is a true-believer, very ideological, and a violent extremist. He is serious about his ideological goals and wants to accomplish them. To do so, he is willing to hide some of his means to accomplish them. For Khamenei, compromise with the U.S., which would lead to stopping the efforts to spread Islamic fundamentalism in the region and overthrowing pro-U.S. regimes, is abandoning the ideals of the revolution. Therefore, Khamenei strongly condemns those who call for rapprochement with the U.S. as selling out the ideals of the revolution. For Khamenei, it is the nature of his regime to be Islamic fundamentalist, which means that it is the regime's religious duty to overthrow secular pro-U.S. regimes in the Islamic world as well as to help destroy Israel. Khamenei is not willing to change his beliefs, which he regards as holy, divine, true, and righteous. For Khamenei, in the struggle against the "Great Satan," either he will prevail, or he will die the exalted death of the martyr. Either way, for Khamenei, his place is assured in heaven.

Notes

1. Philip E. Tetlock and Charles B. McGuire, Jr., "Cognitive Perspectives on Foreign Policy," in G. John Ikenberry, ed., *American Foreign Policy: Theoretical Essays*, 5th edition (New York: Pearson, 2005), 484–501.
2. James David Barber, *The Presidential Character: Predicting Performance in the White House*, 4th edition (Englewood Cliffs, NJ: Prentice-Hall, 1992).
3. Daniel Byman and Kenneth M. Pollack, "Let Us Now Praise Great Men: Bringing the Statesman Back in," *International Security*, vol. 25 (2001): 107–146.
4. Margaret G. Hermann, "Assessing Leadership Style: A Trait Analysis," available at http://www.perceptionmetrics.net/docs/LTA.pdf (accessed December 20, 2012).
5. Alexander George, "The 'Operational Code': A Neglected Approach to the Study of Political Leaders and Decision Making," in G. John Ikenberry, ed., *American Foreign Policy: Theoretical Essays* (New York: HarperCollins, 1989), 483–506.
6. Ali Khamenei, "Biography of the Life of His Eminence Ayatollah Khamenei, the Leader of the Islamic Republic of Iran," (n.d.), available at http://english.khamenei.ir//index.php?option=com_content&task=view&id=57&Itemid=20, (accessed September 20, 2012); Khamenei, "Negahi Gozara Beh Zendeginameh Hazrat Ayatollah Uzma Seyyed Ali Husseini Khamenei" [A Brief Biography of His Eminence Grand Ayatollah Seyyed Ali Husseini Khamenei], (n.d.), in the Persian section at http://farsi.khamenei.ir/memory-content?id=5467, (accessed February 4, 2013). The Persian and English versions are not fully the same; Morad Veysi, "Zendegi Nameh Ayatollah Khamenei" [Biography of Ayatollah Khamenei], Radio Farda, multiple parts (March 31, 2012 through February 2013), available at http://www.radiofarda.com/author/22130.html (accessed August 9, 2012 to February 17, 2013); and Karim Sadjadpour, *Reading Khamenei: The World View of Iran's Most Powerful Leader* (Washington, DC: Carnegie Endowment for International Peace, 2008).

7. Veysi, Part 1.

8. Veysi, Part 2. Tehrani was one of the most radical opponents of the Shah. He initially supported the revolution and was elected to the Assembly of Experts. However, he soon became an opponent of Khomeini, called for the overthrow of the regime, and went to Iraq during the Iran–Iraq War.

9. Khamenei, "Negahi Gozara."

10. "Interview with Mrs. Khamenei," *Mahjubah, The Magazine for Muslim Women*, vol. 100–101 (September–October 1992): 25–26, available at http://www.islam-pure.de/imam/others/others1992.htm, (accessed February 2, 2013).

11. "Interview with Mrs. Khamenei"; and Maziar Radmanesh, "Seyyed Mojtaba Khamenei Kist?" [Who Is Seyyed Mojtaba Khamenei?], originally published at *Rooz Online* July 4, 2009, republished at *Gooya News*, July 5, 2009, available at http://news.gooya.com/politics/archives/2009/07/090353.php (accessed July 5, 2009).

12. Radmanesh, "Seyyed Mojtaba Khamenei Kist?"; and Akbar Alami, "Peyvandhay Famili Baazi Az Maghamat Va Ashkhas Siasi Dar Jomhuri Islami" [Family Connections of Some of the Officials and Personalities in the Islamic Republic], available at http://www.akbaralami.com/Public/ContentBody.aspx?ContentID=3177 (accessed November 12, 2009).

13. Radmanesh, "Seyyed Mojtaba Khamenei Kist?"

14. Veysi, Part 3; and Khamenei, "Biography of the Life."

15. Khamenei, "Biography of the Life."

16. Navab Safavi was his *nom de guerre*. His real name was Seyyed Mojtaba Mir-Lowhi.

17. Homa Katouzian, *Musaddiq and the Struggle for Power in Iran* (London: I.B. Tauris, 1990), 160–161; Ebrahim Norouzi and Arash Norouzi, "Iran's Decade of Assassinations 1946–1955," The Mossadegh Project, January 13, 2011, available at http://www.mohammadmossadegh.com/news/irans-decade-of-assassinations/ (accessed January 16, 2013). There is a lot of evidence that although Khalil Tahmasebi, of the Fadaian Islam, shot Prime Minister Razmara, the bullet that killed Razmara was shot by another assassin under the direction of Mohammad Reza Shah Pahlavi and his man Asadollah Alam. See Katouzian, 83–84.

18. Mashregh News, "Bazgasht Rasmi Fadaian Islam Beh Siasat" [The Official Return of the Fadaian Islam to Politics], November 20, 2011, available at http://www.mashreghnews.ir/fa/print/80153 (accessed February 2, 2013). Abd-Khodae shot Fatemi in the stomach. Fatemi was badly injured but doctors were able to save his life.

19. Mehdi Khalaji, *Apocalyptic Politics: On the Rationality of Iranian Politics* (Washington, DC: Washington Institute for Middle East Policy, 2008), available at http://www.washingtoninstitute.org/pubPDFs/PolicyFocus79Final.pdf (accessed January 5, 2011).

20. Ervand Abrahamian, *Khomeinism: Essays on the Islamic Republic* (Berkeley, CA: University of California Press, 1993), 9.

21. Abrahamian, *Khomeinism*, 9.

22. Abrahamian, *Khomeinism*.

23. Veysi, Part 4; and Khamenei, "Biography of the Life."

24. Veysi, Part 5.

25. Veysi, Part 4.

26. Hussein Ali Montazeri, "Aghay Khamenei Hagh Ham Nadareh Fatwa Bedeh" [Mr. Khamenei Does Not Have the Right to Issue Fatwa], You Tube, posted December 20, 2009, available at http://www.youtube.com/watch?v=pahQw9vMHE8 (accessed December 24, 2009).

27. Veysi, Part 5.

28. Khamenei, "Negahi Gozara."

29. Ibid.

30. Hojatolislam Seyyed Mehdi Andarzgoo, "Zanbili Por Az Mohemat" [A Sack Full of Ammunition], *Khamenei.ir*, August 22, 2013, available at http://farsi.khamenei.ir/others-memory?id=20815 (accessed February 23, 2013).

31. The supporters of Forqan carried out the attempted assassination. Forqan was comprised of the supporters of Dr. Ali Shariati. It was an Islamic group which opposed clerical rule. The would-be

assassins were arrested and executed. Some have erroneously attributed the assassination attempt to the PMOI. See Veysi, part 14, available at http://www.radiofarda.com/content/f3_alikhamenei_bio/24818468.html.

32. Mohammad Ali Aminrad, "Hozor Ayatollah Khamenei Dar Roozhay Moshakbaran Dezful" [Ayatollah Khamenei's Presence at Dezful during the Rains of Rockets], *Khamenei.ir*, May 24, 2013, available at http://farsi.khamenei.ir/others-memory?id=19922 (accessed February 23, 2013).

33. Khamenei, "Biography of the Life"; and Kadmanesh, "Seyyed Mojtaba Khamenei Kist?"

34. Masoud Kazemzadeh, "Foreign Policy Decision Making in Iran," in Valerie Hudson and Klaus Brummer, eds., *Foreign Policy Analysis Beyond North America* (forthcoming).

35. Hussein Bastani, "Afsaneh va Vaghiyat Dar Mored 'Mard Posht Pardeh' Dowlat Ahmadinejad" [Myth and Reality on the 'Man behind the Scenes' of Ahmadinejad's Government], *BBC*, September 16, 2012, available at http://www.bbc.co.uk/persian/iran/2012/09/120916_l39_analysis_khamenei_mashaei_ahmadinejad.shtml (accessed September 18, 2012).

36. Ali Khamenei, "Supreme Leader's Speech to Government Officials," July 24, 2012, available at http://english.khamenei.ir//index.php?option=com_content&task=view&id=1655&Itemid=4 (accessed July 29, 2012).

37. IAEA, Report by the Director General, *Implementation of the NPT Safeguards Agreement and Relevant Provisions of Security Council Resolutions in the Islamic Republic of Iran*, November 8, 2011, available at http://www.iaea.org/Publications/Documents/Board/2011/gov2011–65.pdf (accessed December 20, 2011), especially p. 8.

38. Scott Peterson, "Inside the Mind of Iran's Khamenei," *The Christian Science Monitor*, December 4, 2012, available at http://www.csmonitor.com/World/Middle-East/2012/1204/Inside-the-mind-of-Iran-s-Khamenei-video (accessed December 10, 2012).

39. Ali Akbar Rafsanjani, "Mosahebeh ba Ayatollah Hashemi Rafsanjani: Vakavi Roykardha dar Howzeh Siasat Khareji" [Interview with Ayatollah Hashemi Rafsanjani: Analyzing Viewpoints on the Realm of Foreign Policy], interview by Mahmoud Vaezi and Abbas Maleki, *Rahbord*, vol. 27 (Spring 1382) [Spring 2003]: 5–30.

40. You Tube, "Monazereh Shariatmadari va Asgharzadeh" [Debate between Shariatmadari and Asgharzadeh], posted November 2, 2012, available at http://www.youtube.com/watch?v=-vd0oWeZT94& (accessed November 4, 2012). The debate was held on Iran's state television, and lasted one hour and 54 minutes. Ebrahim Asgharzadeh was the number-two leader of the fundamentalist students who planned, organized, and attacked the U.S. Embassy in Tehran on November 4, 1979, and held 52 Americans hostage for 444 days. Asgharzadeh is a reformist member of the fundamentalist oligarchy. Shariatmadari closely reflects the views of Khamenei.

41. You Tube, "Monazereh Shariatmadari va Asgharzadeh," (author's translation).

42. Ali Khamenei, "Pasokh Rahbar Enghelab Beh 10 Porsesh Dar Bareh Mobarezeh Tarikhi Mellat Iran Ba America" [The Answers of the Leader of the Revolution to 10 Questions on the Historical Struggles of the Iranian People with America], December 6, 2012, available at http://farsi.khamenei.ir/speech-content?id=21721 (accessed February 24, 2013).

43. Ibid.

44. Ibid.

45. Ibid.

46. Ibid.

47. Khamenei, "Supreme Leader's Speech to Government Officials"; and You Tube, "Monazereh Shariatmadari va Asgharzadeh."

48. Ali Khamenei, "Bayanat Dar Haram Mottahar Razavi Dar Avalin Rooz Sale 1392" [Speech at the Shrine of the 8th Imam on the First Day of the Year 1392], March 21, 2013, available at http://farsi.khamenei.ir/speech-content?id=22233 (accessed March 24, 2013).

49. Ibid.

50. Ali Khamenei, "Bayanat Dar Didar Mardom Azaerbaijan" [Speech at the Meeting with the People of Azerbaijan], February 16, 2013, available at http://farsi.khamenei.ir/speech-content?id=22042 (accessed February 17, 2013, author's translation).

51. UN Secretary-General Ban Ki-moon believes that Khamanei is stalling in order for Iran to complete its nuclear weapons. Anne Gearan, "Iran Could Use U.N. Talks as Cover to

Build Bomb, Ban Ki-moon Says," *The Washington Post*, February 14, 2013, available at http://articles.washingtonpost.com/2013–02–14/world/37097672_1_uranium-stockpile-nuclear-program-nuclear-watchdog (accessed February 15, 2013).

52. Mehdi Perpinchi, "Cheragh Sabz Eslah-talabha Dar Vaziyat Ghermez Hastehee" [Green Light of the Reformists under the Red Nuclear Condition], *BBC*, July 18, 2012, available at http://www.bbc.co.uk/persian/iran/2012/07/120718_ll_iran_politics.shtml (accessed July 19, 2012).

53. Khamenei, "Supreme Leader's Speech to Government Officials."

54. Kasra Naji, *Ahmadinejad: The Secret History of Iran's Radical Leader* (Berkeley: University of California Press, 2008); Masoud Kazemzadeh, "Shia Theology, Shia Fundamentalist Ideology, and Mutual Assured Destruction," (forthcoming); Kazemzadeh, "Ahmadinejad's Foreign Policy," *Comparative Studies of South Asia, Africa and the Middle East*, vol. 27 (2007): 423–449; Mahmoud Ahmadinejad, "Speech: U.S. Worried About Emam Zaman," (May 2008), available at http://www.iranian.com/main/singlepage/2008/u-s-worried-about-emam-zaman (accessed June 1, 2008); and *Al Arabiya*, "Ahmadinejad Says US Planning to Prevent Coming of Mahdi: US Wants to Stop Mankind's Savior: Iran Leader," December 7, 2009, available at http://www.alarabiya.net/articles/2009/12/07/93422.html (accessed November 10, 2010); and Golnaz Esfandiari, "Zionists Waiting to Kill Hidden Imam, Says Iranian Cleric," *Radio Free Europe/ Radio Liberty*, September 1, 2010, available at http://www.rferl.org/content/Zionists_Waiting_To_Kill_Hidden_Imam_Says_Iranian_Cleric/2145806.html (accessed November 10, 2010); ISNA, "Saeedi: Sepah Yaki Az Abzarhay Zamineh Saz Zohor Imam Zaman (Aj) Ast" [Saeedi: The IRGC is One of the Instruments for the Creation of Conditions for the Appearance of the 12th Imam], July 27, 2012, available at http://isna.ir/fa/news/91050603505 (accessed July 27, 2012); Tabnak, "Ahmadinejad: Sanad Darim America Mikhahad Joloyeh Zohour Imam Zaman Ra Begirad" [Ahmadinejad: We Have Document on the U.S. Wanting to Prevent the Appearance of the 12th Imam], December 4, 2009, available at http://www.tabnak.ir/fa/pages/?cid=75711 (accessed December 5, 2010); and You Tube, "CIA and MI6 Torture to Get Information on the Hidden Imam Zamaan In Iraq," (2011), program produced by the Iranian state television, posted March 18, 2011, available at http://www.youtube.com/watch?v=mkWT0fcSfg8 (accessed March 20, 2011).

55. Peterson, "Inside the Mind of Iran's Khamenei." On Jamkaran, see its official website at http://www.jamkaran.ir/ (accessed January 19, 2013).

56. Rouholamin Saeedi, "Enghelabiyn Farsoodeh Va Toteeh Jam Zahr" [Dilapidated Revolutionaries and the Conspiracy of Chalice of Poison], *Kayhan*, December 8, 2012, available at http://www.kayhannews.ir/910918/8.htm#other601 (accessed December 10, 2012).

57. Kamran Scot Aghaie, *The Martyrs of Karbala: Shi'i Symbols and Rituals in Modern Iran* (Seattle: WA: University of Washington Press, 2004), 134. Translation and comments in brackets are by Aghaie. "Hoseyn" is another form of spelling of "Hussein." Ali Akbar is Imam Hussein's son.

Hassan Rouhani's Election and Its Consequences for American Foreign Policy

Masoud Kazemzadeh

ABSTRACT Iran is ruled by an oligarchy, thus intra-elite struggles and the evolution of the positions of the supreme leader and the president matter greatly in Iran's foreign policy decision process. This study analyzes the powers of the two decision makers. Then, it presents a detailed analysis of Rouhani's foreign policy orientation. Finally, the article discusses the challenges for American foreign policy presented by Rouhani's election.

The election of Hassan Rouhani to the presidency of Iran in June 2013 raises a number of questions. Why did Supreme Leader Ali Khamenei allow Rouhani to win? What are the consequences of Rouhani's presidency for American foreign policy?

EVOLUTION OF POWER: SUPREME LEADER AND PRESIDENT

Iran is ruled by an oligarchy comprising fundamentalist clerics and laypersons; it is not a one-man dictatorship. Divided by social class, policy preferences, and individual ambition for power, the oligarchy is not and has never been very cohesive. The relative power of various institutional positions, factions, and individuals has fluctuated since the revolution in 1979. All fundamentalist factions (with the partial exception of Ayatollah Hussein Ali Montazeri and his supporters) were fully subservient to Grand Ayatollah Ruhollah Khomeini, the first supreme leader. However, many members of the oligarchy have refused to support the decisions of Ali Khamenei, the second and current supreme leader.

For many years, Khamenei did not exercise the powers granted to the position of supreme leader by the constitution. Between 1989 and 1997, actual power was exercised by Akbar Hashemi Rafsanjani, who was president.[1] The first turning point came in 1997, when Rafsanjani's attempt to change the constitution to allow him to serve a third consecutive term was defeated by other members of the oligarchy, including Khamenei.[2] Those who supported changing the constitution included Hassan Rouhani, Ataollah Mohajerani (Rafsanjani's deputy president for legal and parliamentary affairs), and Seyyed Hussein Marashi (brother-in-law of Rafsanjani and spokesman for Rafsanjani's party: Kargozaran Sazandegi).[3] The election in 1997 brought to power the reformist Mohammad Khatami. His presidency witnessed Khamenei's success in exercising the powers that the constitution had granted the position of supreme leader. Before Khatami's presidential term was over, Khamenei was able to exercise powers beyond those enumerated in the constitution—although Khamenei was not demanding any powers that had not previously been exercised by Khomeini. In fact, Khatami had faithfully submitted to all the actions of Khomeini, including many that were not authorized by the constitution—for example, dismissing Ayatollah Montazeri as the next supreme leader. Articles 107 and 111 of the constitution vest the power to appoint, supervise, and remove a supreme leader in the Assembly of Experts. Thus, Khomeini did not have the constitutional right to choose the next supreme leader; however, about four months before he died, Khomeini simply wrote a letter and dismissed Montazeri. Khatami, Mir-Hossein Moussavi, Mehdi Karrubi, and other reformist members of the oligarchy fully accepted Khomeini's action even though the constitution specifically granted such power to another body. Many believe that behind the scenes Rafsanjani and Khamenei orchestrated the dismissal.[4] From the early years of Khatami's presidency until the present, the actual powers of the supreme leader have been greatly expanded.

Not only the constitution but also unwritten rules strictly circumscribe the powers of the president. The constitution is poorly designed and is unclear about how executive powers over issues such as defense, foreign policy, intelligence, internal security, and culture are divided between the supreme leader and the president. Article 110 specifies some of the powers of the supreme leader, including: (1) delineation of grand policies for the regime; (2) supervision of the execution of the grand policies; (3) commander in chief of all armed forces, for example, the Islamic Revolutionary Guards Corps (IRGC), paramilitary Basij, regular armed forces, and the police; (4) declaration of war and peace; (5) appointment and dismissal of the head of the judicial branch, the six clerical members of the Council of Guardians, the head of the state radio and television monopoly, the head of the IRGC, the head of the regular military, the chairman of the joint chiefs of all armed forces; and (6) dismissal of the president after a vote of the Majles (parliament) or a decision of the high court.

The constitution gives the president the power to nominate his cabinet (Articles 133–137), but the Majles must confirm them (Article 87). Moreover, the Majles has the right to question, impeach, and remove cabinet members (Article 88). The Majles can also question the president. It is widely believed that an arrangement has been agreed to between the president and the supreme leader that, for several sensitive cabinet posts, the president must get the consent of the supreme leader before he submits his nominations to the Majles. These are: foreign minister, defense minister, minister of intelligence, minister of culture and Islamic guidance, and interior minister (a powerful position that oversees elections, appoints governors and deputy governors of the provinces, as well as coordinates with the police concerning security). Although the president appoints the secretary of the Supreme National Security Council (SNSC), which is not a cabinet position and does not require Majles confirmation, he should get the consent of the supreme leader before making the appointment.[5] The supreme leader may even suggest a person for a cabinet post—as occurred in the case of Ataollah Mohajerani for minister of culture and Islamic guidance. Sometimes the negotiations may be long; Dorri Najafabadi was reportedly the fourteenth person that Khatami had suggested for the post of minister of intelligence.[6]

Today, sensitive foreign, defense, and security policies are crafted primarily by the supreme leader with input from his senior advisers, the leadership of the IRGC, and the SNSC. The president and his cabinet are expected to carry out those policies. The president and "his" team (i.e., foreign minister, defense minister, minister of intelligence, interior minister, and secretary of SNSC) do get to be at the table at the SNSC and have a hearing on their policy proposals. The head of the IRGC and the chairman of the joint chiefs of all the armed forces are also members of the SNSC as are two representatives of the supreme leader (Article 176). The SNSC sends its recommendations to the supreme leader, who may or may not accept them. Only if the supreme leader accepts the SNSC's recommendations are they then state policy. In sum, because of how the structures of power have evolved in

Iran, today, the president has a very limited sphere of influence and power while the supreme leader has great power.

INTRA-ELITE FACTIONALISM

The fundamentalist oligarchy is divided into three main factions: hard-liners, expedients, and reformists. Hard-liners (also known as "traditional right" and "*Osolgarayan*" [Principlists]) are divided into various sub-factions—ultra-hard-liners, traditional hard-liners, and moderate hard-liners. Ultra-hard-liners are further divided into three sub-sub-factions: supporters of Khamenei, supporters of Mahmoud Ahmadinejad, and supporters of Ayatollah Mohammad Taghi Mesbah Yazdi (known as "*Jebhe Paydari*" [Steadfast Front]). Khamenei and the ultra-hard-liners are ideologues: they do not want power for the sake of power, they want power so that they can advance their aggressive expansionist policies. They want to expel the United States from the Middle East, eliminate Israel, and establish fundamentalist or friendly regimes in the region. They consider jihad, war, and violence to be part of their ideology.[7]

The expedient faction (also known as "modern right" and "*Kargozaran*" [Executives]) comprises supporters of Ayatollah Rafsanjani—one of the main pillars of the system since 1979. They promote what is called the "Chinese model": modern capitalist IMF-style economic policies, helping the capitalists with tax and other state subsidies for production, détente with the United States, entente with Europe, and maintaining friendly relations with China and Russia. Until 2009, most members of this faction strongly opposed political liberalization and strongly supported political repression. However, in the 2009 election, many leaders of this faction, including its leader Rafsanjani, supported either Mir Hussein Moussavi or Mehdi Karrubi and remained loyal to them during the post-election protests.

Hassan Rouhani has been among the most authoritarian and conservative members of the expedient faction. Between December 2009 and early 2013, he was among the very few members of this faction who remained very close to the supreme leader. From December 2009, Rouhani supported the violent repression of the Green Movement. One constant in Rouhani's long tenure as a high-ranking member of the oligarchy has been his lack of concern about freedoms, democracy, and human rights. For example, in 1999, he was the secretary of SNSC, which formulates domestic and foreign security policy. Also, during the presidential debate held on June 7, 2013, Rouhani presented himself as defending the rights of the student protesters. The hard-line Fars News service published the full text of the speech Rouhani made at the rally of regime supporters on July 14, 1999, following the violent suppression by the IRGC, Basij, and Ministry of Intelligence of the July 9 pro-democracy student sit-in and protests.[8] In the speech, Rouhani viciously insulted the pro-democracy students and praised the Basij, IRGC, Ministry of Intelligence, and others who participated in the violence.

Almost all the reformists (under the guidance and leadership of Khatami) supported Rouhani for president in 2013; almost all the major pro-democracy opposition groups and intellectuals boycotted the election. Only during the 2013 presidential campaign did Rouhani turn his attention to and embrace concerns about political rights.[9] At age 64, whether this concern is genuine or simply a tactic to gain votes from the vast disaffected part of the populace remains to be seen.

The reformist faction of the fundamentalist oligarchy was called the "left faction" between 1979 and 1997. Most of the leaders of the fundamentalist students who stormed the U.S. embassy and took Americans hostage for 444 days were left faction members. The top three leaders were Habibollah Bitaraf, Ibrahim Asgharzadeh, and Mohsen Mirdamadi.[10] Bitaraf became minister of power in Khatami's cabinet during his two terms (1997–2005) as president. Mirdamadi served as a senior adviser to Mir Hussein Moussavi and is currently secretary-general of the Islamic Iran Participation Front, the main reformist party. Other top leaders of the hostage takers were Saeed Hajjarian, Mohsen Aminzadeh, Mohammad Reza Khatami, Masoumeh Ebtekar, and Abbas Abdi.[11] Hajjarian became one the founders of the Ministry of Intelligence and its deputy minister in the 1980s. In the 1990s, he became the main theoretician of the reform movement and a senior adviser to President Khatami. Aminzadeh was named the deputy foreign minister during Khatami's two terms; later, he served as foreign policy adviser to Moussavi. Mohammad

Reza Khatami is the younger brother of President Khatami. The younger Khatami is the former secretary-general of the Islamic Iran Participation Front and is currently one of its top leaders. Masoumeh Ebtekar was the spokeswoman for the hostage taker known as "Mary."[12] She served as deputy to the president on environmental affairs and director of the Environmental Protection Organization under Khatami. President Rouhani appointed her to the same positions. Abdi has been foreign policy adviser to Karrubi.

Members of the left fundamentalist faction, the most dictatorial, anti-American, violent, extremist faction among the fundamentalists, were peacefully purged from positions of power by Rafsanjani and Khamenei in 1992. In 1982, after the Israeli invasion of Lebanon, some of their top leaders (e.g., Ayatollah Ali Akbar Mohtashami-pour, Iran's ambassador to Syria at the time, who helped create the Lebanese Hezbollah as well as serving as interior minister in the 1980s) advocated going to war with Israel, a plea that Khomeini denied. A senior adviser to Moussavi, Mohtashami-pour served as the chair of Moussavi's presidential campaign's "Committee to Safeguard the Votes" in 2009.[13] In 1990, after Iraq, under Saddam Hussein, invaded Kuwait, many left fundamentalists advocated siding with Hussein in the war against the United States.

The left fundamentalists have evolved somewhat; since 1997, they have styled themselves "reformist." Although they still support the highly anti-democratic fundamentalist constitution and its principle of *Velayat Faqih*, they also advocate reduction of political repression, reduction of cultural repression, reduction of social restrictions, and détente with the United States. They have become highly critical of Khamenei's leadership, which they say endangers the preservation of the rule by the fundamentalist oligarchy. The reformists strongly support Khomeini's actions and vigorously defend their own roles during the repression and dictatorship during the 13 years between 1979 and 1992. Khatami, Moussavi, and Karrubi are among the top leaders of the reformist faction.

Between June 2009 and May 2013, within the Green Movement, many reformists worked with the pro-democracy opposition forces—although the relationship was always tense. Whereas the reformists want minor reforms in order to preserve and prolong the system of *Velayat Faqih*, the pro-democracy forces want to replace the current system with a democratic and secular republic. The demands and slogans of the two groups differed greatly. For example, the pro-democracy forces used demands and slogans against the system such as "*Marg bar Asl Velayat Faqih*" (Death to the Principle of Rule of the Cleric); "*Esteghlal, Azadi, Jomhuri Irani*" (Independence, Freedom, Iranian Republic); and "*Naa Sharqi, Naa Gharbi, Jomhuri Irani*" (Neither Eastern, Nor Western, Iranian Republic). The term "Iranian Republic" is used in contradistinction to the "Islamic Republic."

THE 2013 PRESIDENTIAL ELECTION

The supreme leader's authority has come under massive assault since the 2009 election, with protests by reformists, pro-democracy activists, and other opposition groups. Moreover, Ahmadinejad's refusal to fully obey all of Khamenei's wishes since 2010 has further undermined Khamenei. Most significant, the highly effective European and American economic sanctions begun in July 2012 in response to Iran's nuclear program have greatly undermined Iran's economy and have galvanized opposition to Khamenei's foreign policies.

The ultra-hard-line Khamenei has opposed granting major concessions to the P5+1 (five permanent members of the UN Security Council plus Germany) in the nuclear negotiations, opposed holding bilateral negotiations with the United States to resolve differences between the two countries, opposed Israeli–Palestinian peace agreements based on a two-state solution, and has supported providing military, economic, and political assistance to President Bashar al-Assad of Syria.[14] Ultra-hard-liners argue that Iranians should bear the difficulties of the sanctions to resist the demands of the United States. Saeed Jalili, Iran's former chief nuclear negotiator and former secretary of the SNSC, belongs to this group. During the campaign for president, Jalili was the closest to Khamenei.

By allowing Rouhani and Mohammad Reza Aref (first deputy president to Khatami) to compete in the June 2013 presidential election, Khamenei succeeded in convincing the expedients and reformists to go to the polls. The cooperation between the democratic opposition forces and the reformists in the aftermath of the 2009 election had greatly threatened the stability of the regime. The regime became far more secure after the 2013 election because it had been able to bring the reformists back into the political life of the country.

Khamenei could not have easily manipulated the 2013 election for three main reasons. First, the hard-line camp was bitterly divided, with four major candidates; thus, to manipulate the process and the result in favor of one candidate would have badly alienated the other candidates and their supporters. Second, much of the state apparatus responsible for the election was in the hands of Ahmadinejad's loyalists in the Ministry of Interior and provincial governors—who were upset that their candidate had been disqualified by the Council of Guardians. Third, some powerful moderate hard-liners (e.g., Ali Akbar Nategh Nouri and Ali Mottahari) openly and strongly supported Rouhani. Ali Akbar Velayati was the candidate of both the traditional hard-liners and the moderate hard-liners. Many other moderate hard-liners (e.g., Speaker of Majles Ali Larijani, Deputy Speaker of Majles Mohammad Reza Bahonar, and member of Majles Ahmad Tavakoli) appeared to prefer Rouhani over both Jalili and Mohammad Bagher Ghalibaf. The first choice of traditional hard-liners and many moderate hard-liners was Velayati, however, they were even more strongly opposed to Jalili and Ghalibaf. For example, some in the Council of Guardians opposed the ultra-hard-liners and also opposed the disqualification of Rafsanjani and Rouhani. Ayatollah Mahmoud Hashemi Shahroudi may be among this group. Those in the Council of Guardians sympathetic to Rafsanjani and Rouhani leaked the confidential proceedings to the reformist and expedient camps, while the hard-line members leaked this information to the hard-line camps.[15]

The election of either Jalili or Gholam-Ali Haddad Adel (father-in-law of Khamenei's politically ambitious son Mojtaba), both of whom fully agree with Khamenei and are completely subservient to him, would have best served the interests of the supreme leader. Jalili had the enthusiastic support of the ultra-hard-liners as well as much of the Basij rank and file. Some in the IRGC rank and file may also have supported him. During the presidential debates, Jalili and Haddad Adel fully supported and defended the policies associated with the supreme leader. Adel withdrew from the race several days before the election as it became clear that his support was in the low single digits.

Rouhani does not pose a serious threat to Khamenei's power and has repeatedly reassured the supreme leader and the hard-line camp of his loyalty. According to Mohammad Reza Bahonar, the deputy speaker of the Majles, "about 7 or 8 days before the election, Mr. Rouhani wrote a letter to the esteemed Supreme Leader and reiterated that he had always been obedient and cooperative with him and would remain so."[16] In contrast, the leading hard-line candidate, Gen. Mohammad Bagher Ghalibaf, might have posed a serious threat to Khamenei.

Ghalibaf had been a highly competent commander of the IRGC during the Iraq–Iran war (1980–1981). He was the commander of the IRGC's air force, head of the national police, and, since 2005, had served as mayor of Tehran, a city of more than 10 million. Large numbers of IRGC generals headed Ghalibaf's election teams around the country and were a large part of his campaign. Gen. Ghasem Soleymani, the commander of the Qods Force, the elite foreign operations force of the IRGC, was also said to strongly support Ghalibaf.[17] Soleymani is highly popular among the IRGC leadership and rank and file. Ghalibaf is unusually competent and highly ambitious. In July 1999, Ghalibaf and Soleymani co-authored a confidential threatening letter (co-signed by about two dozen high-ranking IRGC commanders) to then-president Khatami warning him that if he could not restore calm to university campuses during the pro-democracy protests, the IRGC would take matters into its own hands. This letter, which was published by the ultra-hard-line *Kayhan* daily, was the first time that the IRGC had entered national politics in such a manner. The supreme leader not only did not discipline Ghalibaf and the IRGC commanders, he promoted Ghalibaf to head of the national police. With the support of the IRGC, from 1999 onward, Khamenei began a massive struggle to undermine and contain Khatami's power.

In the 2005 presidential race, Ghalibaf was the front runner among the hard-liners until he said that he would become the "Hezbollah version of Reza Shah." Reza Shah was a competent military commander who carried out a coup in February 1921 and made himself the supreme commander of the armed forces. Shortly thereafter, Reza made himself minister of defense and then prime minister; in January 1926, he established his own dynasty. Like Reza Shah, Ghalibaf presents authoritarian military solutions to political uncertainties and chaos. Soon after the comment, Khamenei's support moved from Ghalibaf to Ahmadinejad.

After Ahmadinejad's ascendance to the presidency in 2005, the political and economic power of the IRGC grew tremendously, causing concern among many members of the oligarchy, including some moderate hard-liners. A Ghalibaf victory in the 2013 presidential elections would have greatly increased IRGC's power and dramatically changed the balance of power. Today. Khamenei can control the IRGC; however, had Ghalibaf become president and serious conflicts over policies were to arise between the two, Khamenei almost certainly would have lost control of the IRGC. Moreover, concerns have been expressed that after Khamenei's death, the IRGC commanders might interfere with the selection process in the Assembly of Experts. What is also not clear is would IRGC commanders remain subservient to a supreme leader, whom they do not like.

Right before the election, Khamenei issued a memorandum to the armed forces and the *Imaman Jomeh* (leaders of Friday prayers). The *Imaman Jomeh* are appointed by Khamenei and are considered to be the most powerful man or men in each town; the letter instructed them not to support any candidate.[18] On the one hand, this memorandum prevented the conflicts among the supporters of the hard-line candidates from turning into internecine conflicts among various factions within the IRGC, Basij, and the *Imaman Jomeh*. On the other hand, the lack of mobilization of the voters by the IRGC, Basij, and the *Imaman Jomeh* forestalled the mass vote on behalf of the hard-line candidates. With no hard-line institution to mobilize rural and small-town voters, large numbers of them voted for Rouhani. Historically such votes had gone to the hard-line candidates in both presidential and parliamentary elections.[19]

ROUHANI'S FOREIGN POLICY

After the revolution, Rouhani was elected to the Majles and served five four-year terms between 1980 and 2000, rising to become deputy Majles speaker during the fourth (1992–1996) and fifth (1996–2000) terms; during these same two terms he also served as chairman of the Foreign Policy Committee. Earlier in his tenure at the Majles he was chairman of the Defense Committee (first and second terms). For several years during the Iran–Iraq war, Khomeini delegated his power as commander in chief to Rafsanjani; Rouhani served as deputy to Rafsanjani at that time. Since the establishment of SNSC in 1989, Rouhani has been one of the two representatives of the supreme leader to the SNSC. Rouhani was chosen to serve as secretary of the SNSC from 1989 to 2005 under presidents Rafsanjani and Khatami; he has also been the national security adviser to both these presidents. Rouhani's experience includes ongoing service as a member of the Assembly of Experts since 1999 and a member of the Expediency Council since 1991.[20] Competently filling these positions would make Rouhani one of the top 40, if not one of the top 20, most powerful members of the oligarchy between 1981 and 2005. With the rise of the ultra-hard-liners in 2005, expedient and reformist members of the oligarchy lost top positions of power. Between 2005 and May 2013, Rouhani was probably among the top 100 (but not top 40) members of the oligarchy.

Since 1992, Rouhani has been the director of the Expediency Council's think tank, the Center for Strategic Research, which conducts research for that body.[21] Another responsibility of the Expediency Council is to formulate long-term general policies and strategies for Iran's economy, foreign policy, and security; these general policies are submitted to the supreme leader for ratification.

When Iran's clandestine nuclear program was exposed in 2002, the heads of the various branches of the state decided to choose one person to be in charge and chose the urbane and sophisticated Rouhani whose public pronouncements sound rational and pragmatic.

While Rouhani is a centrist or moderate within the fundamentalist ruling oligarchy, he is decidedly not a centrist or moderate in Iranian politics. In Iranian politics, the main centrist or moderate parties are the Iran National Front (founded by Dr. Mossadegh in 1949, it is a coalition of liberal democrats and social democrats) and the National Movement of Iranian Resistance (founded by Dr. Shapour Bakhtiar in 1979, it is a highly secular group of democrats).[22] Other groups include the communists on the far left, the monarchists on the right, and the fundamentalists on the far right. Every major party or movement has a mix of extreme and moderate right, left, and center members. For example, in al Qaeda, abu Musab Al-Zarqavi was more right-wing and extreme than Osama bin Laden and Ayman al-Zawahiri. This means that within al Qaeda, bin Laden was moderate and centrist compared to al-Zarqavi. But this does not mean that bin Laden is a centrist or moderate in Saudi Arabia, the Islamic world, or world politics. Within members of the fundamentalist oligarchy, Rouhani is a centrist compared with Khamenei and Ahmadinejad to the right and with Rafsanjani and Khatami to the left.

The Islamic fundamentalist oligarchy is a far right, extremist, reactionary, misogynist, violent, dictatorial group within Iranian politics. Islamic fundamentalists in Iran supported Khomeini, who began his political and religious activities in the early 1940s. In his first booklet, *Kashef al Asrar* (1943), Khomeini (who was an assistant to Grand Ayatollah Brujerdi, the highest-ranking cleric in Iran at the time and a monarchist) was openly and explicitly monarchist and a traditional Shia.[23] After the 1953 coup, Khomeini took secret messages from Brujerdi to the shah.[24] Khomeini remained a monarchist until June 1963. The June 1963 land reform (taking land from big landowners and distributing acreage among the peasants), female enfranchisement, and no longer requiring taking the oath of office on the Qoran (which would have allowed Christians, Jews, Bahais, and Zoroastrians to use their sacred texts to swear an oath and thus to hold high office) made Khomeini oppose the shah and, soon, the system of monarchy.[25] Over the years, Khomeini evolved from an ultra-conservative to a fundamentalist,[26] becoming more reactionary and traditional than the shah and the monarchists.

How does Rouhani explain his policies in private to other members of the oligarchy? He did speak at length (late in 2004; Khatami was president and present) in private to members of the Supreme Council of Cultural Revolution, explaining the rationale for the policies he pursued during the nuclear negotiations. Hard-liners had raised many questions about the wisdom of the agreements that Rouhani had reached in late 2003 and early 2004 with the EU3 (the United Kingdom, France, and Germany). Between March and September 2005, concerns had turned into harsh condemnations of the suspension of the uranium enrichment program and the acceptance of additional protocols. Rouhani decided to respond publicly by publishing the transcripts of the secret talk in the fall 2005 issue of *Rahbord*, the quarterly scholarly journal published by the think tank that Rouhani heads.[27] We can assume that some top-secret material had been deleted from the text and other (false) materials added. For example, had Rouhani said that Iran had a clandestine nuclear weapons program, he would have certainly deleted that and instead inserted the opposite. In his confidential speech, Rouhani explains why he made the agreement. Following is my translation of Rouhani's words:

> From about 15–16 years ago—that is the years 1366–1667 [1987–1988 CE], one of the things that the Islamic Republic of Iran pursued was to achieve [nuclear] fuel cycle technology...
>
> In recent years, that is from 1378 [1999], the decision was made to become more active. For this reason, the work was redoubled...
>
> After these activities [were exposed] in the summer of 1381 [2002], there was talk in the Western media that Iran was working on making an atomic bomb... (8)

> In this meeting, the Europeans [EU3] promised us that if we presented the full picture of the nuclear program to the IAEA, then if the Americans insisted on taking the case to the UN Security Council, they would resist and would not permit that to occur... (13)

> The Europeans did what they promised in the November [2003] meeting [of the IAEA Board of Governors]...
>
> However, later on, the confidence-building between us and the Europeans got into some trouble... Let me add a point here that, at that juncture, we were not aware of the behind-the-scenes negotiations between the U.S., the UK, and Libya. Also, we did not know that the middleman [the interlocutor between the A. Q. Khan network and Iran] from whom we had purchased the [nuclear] equipment was the same middleman from whom the Libyans also bought their materials. In a separate report we wrote a note about the middleman and the materials that we bought from him and, separately and privately, gave it to [Mohamed] El Baradei along with the complete picture of Iran's dossier to the IAEA...
>
> The Libyans had reported the whole thing from the beginning to end to the Americans and the English... (14)

> Anyway, from the intelligence that they had gotten from Libya, they discovered that it is possible that we had gotten other things from the middleman and had not disclosed them. We told them about the materials that we got from

this middleman, except about the P2, which we did not tell them about. And, because they had found out about the middleman from the Libyans, they had gotten to him and had gotten sufficient intelligence . . . (14–15)

Anyway, the P2 case caused harm to the trust between the Europeans and us and it did major harm to the process that we had begun. The Americans from the very first days were telling Europeans that Iranians were telling you lies and have not told you all the things and what they have declared is only part of the whole program. But the Europeans told them that we trust them. When the case of the P2 was discovered, the Europeans got angry and basically questioned whether we had gotten other materials and not disclosed them. For example, they asked us did you also get the design for the atomic bomb? Because Libya had also bought the design for the bomb [from the same source] . . . (16)

Another issue that emerged was that the Europeans gradually reached the decision that we only accepted suspension on those aspects of the technology that we had already mastered and did not accept suspension on those aspects of technology that we still had problems with . . . That is, in Esfehan, during the suspension, we completed the parts of U.C.F. [Uranium Conversion Facility] and the factory that converts yellow cake into UF4 and UF6. At the time that we were talking with the Europeans in Tehran, we were still installing the equipment in some of the places in Esfehan and still a lot more work to finish. In reality, with the calm atmosphere that we created, we managed to finish the projects and, thanks to Allah, today [the projects at] Esfehan have been completed and we can transform yellow cake into UF4 and UF6—this is very significant . . . (16–17)

Perhaps this way we could reach a good accord with the Europeans. Even if we don't reach one, we will negotiate for some months with the Europeans, and, at the end, we will be where we are today; at the minimum, we will postpone our case being referred to the Security Council. If we were supposed to be going to the Security Council, we could postpone this for one more year and finish the work on public opinion and use this opportunity to advance our [nuclear] technology and fix the legal issues with the IAEA . . . (25–26)

We should be patient and find the most appropriate time for breaking the suspension [of uranium enrichment and implementing the additional protocol] . . . (33)

We had hidden many things and thought that no one knew about them, but these things that we had hidden, unfortunately [our scientists] had published the [secret] research in a scholarly article, a master's thesis, and a doctoral dissertation. Some other matters were also disclosed to the IAEA by China and Russia . . .

On the matter of the middleman that was mentioned here, we have never mentioned to them [the IAEA] the word "Pakistan," we only said that we bought it from a middleman. We told them the first person we bought the materials from was from Europe. Then, they said this man called "Taher" that you dealt with, what country is he from? In response, we told them from his looks, he looks like someone from the subcontinent. The name of Pakistan was presented by the IAEA. Of course, as you know, Libya had revealed everything. But we did not say anything. We were considerate of Pakistan, but others revealed the issue and now we are at this point. (34)

In the speech, Rouhani also says that Iran received information on P1, P2, and centrifuge equipment. However, according to the information discovered by the IAEA, the A. Q. Khan network had also provided a nuclear bomb design to Iran. According to the IAEA report: "In an interview in 2007 with a member of the clandestine nuclear supply network, the Agency [IAEA] was told that Iran had been provided with nuclear explosive design information. From information provided to the Agency during that interview, the Agency is concerned that Iran may have obtained more advanced design information than the information identified in 2004 as having been provided to Libya by the nuclear supply network."[28] Either Rouhani deleted this central fact in the published transcript or hid this fact from the members of the oligarchy.

Rouhani is a smart, cunning, pragmatic, and strategic thinker. He considers Israel and the United States to be strategic enemies. He says that the EU, Russia, and China oppose Iran having a full nuclear fuel cycle. He maintains that if Iran is to come out on top, it must separate the EU from the United States; if the United States and the EU stick together, then Russia would not veto the UN Security Council resolutions. The Chinese have great trade relations with the United States and would not jeopardize them with a veto at the Security Council unless the Russians or the EU (e.g., the United Kingdom and France) oppose the United States and would be willing to use their veto. Rouhani also believes that Iran should try to bring South Africa and Brazil into the negotiations because those two countries want to have a full fuel cycle. Rouhani's objectives: avoid and/or delay Iran's case being referred from the IAEA Board of Governors to the UN Security Council in order to avoid sanctions, while preserving Iran's nuclear program. His plan was to deceive the Europeans to buy time for Iran to develop its nuclear program. Once the Europeans found out, Iran would have already overcome the technological hurdles to mastering the full nuclear fuel cycle. Rouhani says that once a country has achieved either completion of the fuel cycle or the building of an atomic bomb, then the world has to accept the fait accompli (as with Pakistan's nuclear bomb and Brazil's full fuel cycle). A country is vulnerable, Rouhani reasoned, only when it is at the doorstep of either mastering the technology for a full fuel cycle or at the beginning of assembling an atomic bomb. Rouhani used diplomacy to give Iran time to complete its nuclear program.

CONSEQUENCES FOR U.S. FOREIGN POLICY

Iran's collapsing economy was one of the main reasons for the unpopularity of the hard-liners; it helped Rouhani get elected. Economic sanctions, especially EU and U.S. sanctions imposed in July 2012 that reduced Iran's ability to sell oil, gravely affected Iran's economy. According to the World Bank's June 2013 report, Iran's compound average annual Gross Domestic Product (GDP) growth rate between 2000 and 2009 was 4.6 percent. The annual GDP growth rate for 2010 was 5.9 percent; for 2011, it was 1.7 percent; and, for 2012, it was −1.9 percent.[29] The same report indicated Iran's year-to-year inflation rate to be over 40 percent, among the three highest in the world.[30]

Many of the sanctions could only be removed if fundamental changes were made to Iran's foreign policy. Initially, Rouhani tried to convince Khamenei to embrace his policy proposals on U.S.–Iran relations, nuclear negotiations with the P5+1, and Syria. The power disparity was simply too great for Rouhani to successfully challenge Khamenei's authority. What was discussed were what policies and tactics would best serve the interests of the Islamic Republic and those of the supreme leader (in the long term at least).

Khamenei had to decide to accept Rouhani's policy changes or refuse them. Khamenei has three options: (1) accept the major changes proposed by Rouhani; (2) reject Rouhani's proposals and then use his enormous powers to contain and undermine Rouhani if Rouhani refused to fully obey his wishes; or (3) reject Rouhani's proposals and then utilize Rouhani's great diplomatic skills to forestall further sanctions and buy time for the nuclear program if Rouhani agreed to cooperate.

We would know that Khamenei accepted Rouhani's policy changes if Iran had agreed to authorize high-level representatives to hold negotiations with the United States to resolve the major differences between the two sides and/or if Iran would propose or accept far-reaching proposals with the P5+1. We would know that Rouhani failed to convince Khamenei to make major changes if such changes were not forthcoming or if Rouhani resigned. We would know that Khamenei decided to utilize Rouhani to carry out his policies and Rouhani agreed to cooperate if, by October or November 2013, only minor and cosmetic changes had been made in foreign policy. Events between July 2013 and January 2014 have clearly shown that Khamenei has accepted Rouhani's policies, at least for the time being. However, what is not clear are the outlines and aims of Khamenei's true strategic and tactical red lines nor is it clear how much time Rouhani has been provided to accomplish their goals.

Time is of essence if Iran has a clandestine nuclear weapons program. Ban Ki-moon, the UN secretary-general, for example, believes that Khamenei has been stalling to give Iran time to complete its nuclear weapons program.[31] Stalling tactics like making or allowing small steps, offering minor proposals, or taking cosmetic measures while allowing the uranium enrichment program to continue give Iran's nuclear scientists the time they need to complete their work. The consensus, as shown by several UN Security Council resolutions, had been that Iran must stop all enrichment-related activities. That consensus was shattered by the November 24, 2013, agreement between the P5+1 and Iran, which allowed Iran to enrich at low levels. By January 2014, Rouhani's policies had succeeded in preventing further sanctions (by the United States, UN, EU) and the rolling back of some existing sanctions while preserving the enrichment program and infrastructure.

The primary goals of Rouhani and the expedient faction are the preservation of the clerical regime and economic development. They are pragmatists willing to compromise to avoid a war with the United States. Khamenei and the ultra-hard-liners are ideologues, with many uncomfortable with Rouhani's policies. In view of the volatility of Iranian politics, Rouhani's position is very fragile. How long his policies can remain viable depends on Khamenei and the power of the hard-line factions.

How Khamenei responds to Rouhani as well as how the United States, the EU, and other members of the P5+1 react to Khamenei's policy will determine whether there will be peace, a war of choice, or a war of necessity.

Notes

1. Ali Akbar Rafsanjani, "*Mosahebeh ba Ayatollah Hashemi Rafsanjani: Vakavi Roykardha dar Howzeh Siasat Khareji*" [Interview with Ayatollah Hashemi Rafsanjani: Analyzing Viewpoints on the Realm of Foreign Policy], interview by Mahmoud Vaezi and Abbas Maleki, *Rahbord* 27 (Spring 1382 [2003]): 5–30.
2. "*Zakani Dar Daneshgah Tehran: Moshkel Jeddi Maa Adam Bologh Kesani Ast Keh Modaii Kohnekari Siasi Hastand*" [Zakani at the University of Tehran: The Serious Problem Here Is the Lack of Maturity among Those Who Claim to Be Old Hands in Politics], ISNA (Iranian Student News Agency, an official state agency), November 22, 2009, http://www.isna.ir/ISNA/NewsView.aspx?ID=News-1444221&Lang=P. Mr. Zakani has been one of the top ultra-hard-line leaders in the Majles.
3. *Ibid.*
4. Neil Shevlin, "Velayat-e Faqih in the Constitution of Iran: The Implementation of Theocracy," *Journal of Constitutional Law* 1, no. 2 (Fall 1998): 375.
5. Arash Bahmani, "*Gamaneh-zani Dar Bareh Dowlat Rouhani: Hamrahan Cabineh 'Tadbir va Omid' Cheh Kesani Hastand*" [Guessing about Rouhani's Government: Who Will Be in the Cabinet of "Wisdom and Hope"], Roozonline, June 20, 2013, http://www.roozonline.com/persian/news/newsitem/archive/2013/june/20/article/-fcf86e7d61.html; "*Rouhani Goruhi Ra 'Masoul Barasi Abad Mozakereh Bah Gorouh 5+1 Kardeh Ast*'" [Rouhani Has Chosen a Group "For Assessing Various Dimensions of the Negotiations with the Group of P5+1"], BBC, June 26, 2013, http://www.bbc.co.uk/persian/iran/2013/06/130626_mgh_iran_rouhani_nuclear.shtml; "*Mokhalefat Khamenei Ba Entekhab Yunesi Beh Onvan Vazir Ettelaat*" [Khamenei's Opposition to the Selection of Yunesi for the Position of Minister of Intelligence], Iran Emrooz, June 28, 2013, http://www.iran-emrooz.net/index.php/news2/46360/.
6. Bahmani, "Guessing About."
7. Masoud Kazemzadeh, "Ayatollah Khamenei's Foreign Policy Orientation," *Comparative Strategy* 32, no. 5 (2013): 443–458; Masoud Kazemzadeh, "Ahmadinejad's Foreign Policy," *Comparative Studies of South Asia, Africa and the Middle East* 27, no. 2 (2007): 423–449.
8. Hassan Rouhani, "*Sokhanrani Hojatolislam Hassan Rouhani Dar Bareh Ashubhay 18 Tir 78*" [Hojatolislam Hassan Rouhani's Speech on the Riots of July 9, 1999], Fars News Agency, June 9, 2013, http://www.farsnews.com/newstext.php?nn=13920319000749.
9. Hassan Rouhani's website, http://rouhani.ir/.
10. YouTube, "*Monazereh Shariatmadari va Asgharzadeh*" [Debate between Shariatmadari and Asgharzadeh], November 2, 2012, http://www.youtube.com/watch?v=-vd0oWeZT94&.
11. "*Mozea Ahmadinejad Dar Bareh Taskhir Laneh Jasusi*" [Ahmadinejad's Position on the Occupation of the Den of Spies], *Farda News*, November 21, 2011, http://www.fardanews.com/fa/news/171597/موضع-احمدی‌نژاد-درباره-تسخیر-لانه-جاسوسی.
12. Elaine Sciolino, "Top Woman in Iran's Government Once Spoke for Hostage-Takers," *New York Times*, January 28, 1998.
13. Shahryar Sadr, "How Hezbollah Founder Fell Foul of Iranian Regime: At Home, Exporter of Islamic Revolution Was Dedicated Reformer—and That Was His Undoing," Institute for War and Peace Reporting, July 8, 2010, http://iwpr.net/report-news/how-hezbollah-founder-fell-foul-iranian-regime; "Mousavi Call for Truth Commission," Press TV, June 17, 2009, http://edition.presstv.ir/detail/98307.html; "Speech by Former Interior Minister Detailing Election Fraud Released," The Green Voice of Freedom, October 12, 2010, http://en.irangreenvoice.com/content/2541.
14. Kazemzadeh, "Ayatollah Khamenei's Foreign Policy Orientation."
15. "*Barrasi Dobareh Selahiyat Hassan Rouhani Dar Jalaseh Shoray Negahban Sehat Dashteh Ast*" [The Second Vetting of Hassan Rouhani at the Meeting of the Council of Guardians Was True], Kaleme, June 27, 2013, http://www.kaleme.com/1392/04/06/klm-149546. Ayatollah Shahroudi is a member of Council of Guardians and the Assembly of Experts. A moderate hard-liner, he is one of three prominent ayatollahs considered possible successors to Khamenei. The others are the ultra-hard-liner Mesbah Yazdi and the expedient Rafsanjani.
16. "*Bahonar: Rouhani Yek Hafteh Pish Az Entekhabat Beh Rahbari Nameh Nevesht*" [Bahonar: Rouhani Wrote a Letter to the Supreme Leader a Week before the Election], Radio Farda, June 23, 2013, http://www.radiofarda.com/content/f12_rouhani_letter_to_khamenei_on_obedience/25025306.html.
17. Karim Sadjadpour, "Nate Silvering the Iranian Elections," *Foreign Policy* online, June 13, 2013, http://www.foreignpolicy.com/articles/2013/06/13/nate_silvering_the_iranian_elections_khamenei.
18. "*Ansari: Rahbari Baray Adam Dekhalat Dar Entekhabat Beh Nirohay Mosalah Bakhshnameh Dadeh Bood*" [Ansari: The Supreme Leader Had Issued a Memorandum to the Armed Forces on Not Interfering in the Election], Radio Farda, June 25, 2013, http://www.radiofarda.com/content/f9_iran_presidential_election_2013_ansari_khameneie/25027808.html.
19. Masoud Kazemzadeh, "Intra-Elite Factionalism and the 2004 Majles Elections in Iran," *Middle Eastern Studies* 44, no. 2 (2008): 189–214.
20. "Hassan Rouhani's Biography," al Alam, June 15, 2013, http://en.alalam.ir/news/1484685. Al Alam is the official Arabic-language satellite television program of the Iranian government.
21. Center for Strategic Research site is at http://www.csr.ir/.
22. Masoud Kazemzadeh, "The Perils and Costs of a Grand Bargain with the Islamic Republic of Iran," *American Foreign Policy Interests* 29, no. 5 (2007): 301–327.
23. Ervand Abrahamian, *Khomeinism: Essays on the Islamic Republic* (Berkeley & Los Angeles: University of California Press, 1993), 9.
24. *Ibid.*, 9.

25. Willem Floor, "The Revolutionary Character of the Iranian Ulama: Wishful Thinking or Reality?," *International Journal of Middle East Studies* 12, no. 1 (December 1980).
26. Abrahamian, *Khomeinism*.
27. Hassan Rouhani, "*Farasoyeh Chaleshhay Iran Va Agance Dar Parvandeh Hastehee*" [Behind the Challenges of Iran and the IAEA in the Nuclear Dossier], *Rahbord* 37 (Fall 1384 [2005]), http://www.csr.ir/center.aspx?lng=fa&abtid=08&centid=41&semid=235.
28. IAEA, *Implementation of the NPT Safeguards Agreement and Relevant Provisions of Security Council Resolutions in the Islamic Republic of Iran* (November 8, 2011), http://www.iaea.org/Publications/Documents/Board/2011/gov2011-65.pdf, Annex, 8.
29. World Bank, *Global Economic Prospects 7* (Washington, DC: June 2013), 175, https://openknowledge.worldbank.org/handle/10986/13892.
30. *Ibid.*, 50.
31. Anne Gearan, "Iran Could Use U.N. Talks as Cover to Build Bomb, Ban Ki-moon Says," *Washington Post*, February 14, 2013, http://articles.washingtonpost.com/2013-02-14/world/37097672_1_uranium-stockpile-nuclear-program-nuclear-watchdog.

The Perils and Costs of a Grand Bargain with the Islamic Republic of Iran

Masoud Kazemzadeh

Abstract

In this article the author presents an analysis of the perils and costs that the United States is likely to incur if it enters into a grand bargain in general with the Islamic Republic of Iran or into a specific grand bargain based on the proposal advanced by Flynt Leverett and Hillary Mann.

Among other factors, the American failure to stabilize Iraq and Afghanistan has fueled Iran's attempt at regional supremacy to the consternation of many in the region and beyond. The failure of the containment policy, fear that the Islamic Republic will develop nuclear weapons, and the bellicose rhetoric and policies of Iran's new president, Mahmoud Ahmadinejad, have given rise to urgent discussions about how best to counter the threat of the fundamentalist regime. The main policies under discussion are regime change; surgical strikes; reconfigured containment; limited, issue-based dialogue; and a "grand bargain."

The most detailed proposal for a grand bargain is articulated by Flynt Leverett and Hillary Mann. Dr. Leverett served as a senior director of Middle East affairs at the National Security Council (NSC), Middle East specialist on the secretary of state's Policy Planning Staff, and a senior analyst at the CIA. He left the NSC in 2003. He is currently a senior fellow at the New America Foundation. Hillary Mann Leverett engaged in extensive negotiations with Iranian officials during her service at the Permanent Mission of the United States to the UN and the National Security Council.

After the White House demanded redaction of parts of their op-ed article for *The New York Times*, much controversy ensued. *The New York Times* published the redacted version of the original op-ed article on December 22, 2006. It is based on a larger study by Leverett entitled "Dealing with Tehran: Assessing U.S. Diplomatic Options Toward Iran," published on December 4.[1] In this article, I present some of the perils and costs of a grand bargain in general and the grand bargain proposed by Leverett and Mann in particular.

The United States previously pursued containment of the fundamentalist regime that came to power in 1979. Initially this was conducted awkwardly via balancing through Iraq, which was closely allied with the Soviet Union and France. Saddam's invasion of Kuwait and the collapse of the Soviet Union allowed the Clinton administration to attempt to contain both Iran and Iraq, a policy aptly named "dual containment." Intermittently there have been attempts at rapprochement with the fundamentalist regime.

President Bush's overthrow of Saddam caused great anxiety among Iran's rulers. Concerned that a similar fate was awaiting them, in May 2003 the supreme leader agreed to send the Bush administration a roadmap, developed by Iran's ambassador to France and the Swiss ambassador to Tehran, to resolve U.S.–Iran differences.[2] Initial reports that the roadmap was initiated by all of the regime officials are false. In addition, the reports that the supreme leader agreed with all of the serious concessions are false as well.

The actual text of the accompanying notes by Swiss Ambassador Tim Guldimann indicates that the roadmap was his brainchild and that of Iran's then Ambassador Sadeq Kharrazi (a nephew of the foreign minister and a former deputy foreign minister, whose sister is married to the supreme leader's son). Moreover, the text states that the supreme leader only agreed with 85 to 90 percent of the proposals. In other words, the supreme leader was opposed to 10 to 15 percent of the proposals. In his fax to the State Department containing the text of the roadmap, Guldimann wrote:

> 1. **On April 21, I had a longer discussion with Sadeq Kharrazi** who came to see me.... **During this discussion a first draft of the enclosed Roadmap was developed.** He said that he would discuss this with the Leader and the Foreign Minister.
>
> 2. **On May 2, I met him again for three hours.** He told me that he had **two long discussions with the Leader on the Roadmap.** In these meetings, which both lasted almost two hours, only President **Khatami** and **FM Kharrazi** were present; "we went through every word of this [sic] paper." (He additionally had a series of separate meetings with both). The question is dealt with in high secrecy, therefore no one else has been informed. (S.Kh. himself has become also very discreet in our last contacts). S. Kh. presented the paper to the Leader **as a proposal which he had discussed 'with a friend in Europe who has close contacts with higher echelons in the DoS';** The Leader explicitly hat [sic] asked him whether this is a US-proposal and S.Kh. denied this, saying that, if it is accepted, this friend could convey it to Washington as the basis for opening the bilateral discussion.
>
> 3. Then S.Kh. told me that the Leader uttered some **reservations** as for some points; the President and the Foreign Minister were very positive, there was no problem from their side. Then he said "They (meaning above all the Leader) agree **with 85%–90% of the paper**. But everything can be negotiated."[3]

The roadmap calls on the fundamentalist regime to stop providing material support to Hamas and Palestinian Islamic Jihad (PIJ) from Iranian territory, put pressure on Hamas and PIJ to stop violence against civilians within 1967 borders, take action on Lebanese Hezbollah to become exclusively a political and social organization within Lebanon, accept the two-state approach, help stabilize Iraq, make the nuclear program transparent, and take decisive action against Al Qaeda in Iranian territory. In exchange, the roadmap asked the Bush administration to give the regime a security guarantee ("The United States will refrain from supporting changes of the political system by direct interference from outside"), respect Iran's interests in Iraq; recognize "Iran's legitimate security interests in the region with the accompanying defense capacity," abolish all sanctions, release Iran's frozen assets, and take "action against MKO and affiliated organizations in the United States." Some of these have been further elaborated as immediate steps such as "U.S. commitment to resolve MKO problem in Iraq" and "Iranian commitment to decisive actions against Al Qaida members in Iran."[4]

A slightly different version of the roadmap has been provided by the fundamentalist regime.[5] In this document the regime spelled out what it meant by "security guarantee." The fundamentalist regime expected the United States to "halt... hostile behavior and rectification of the status of Iran." The U.S. government must make a public statement that the fundamentalist regime "did not belong to 'the axis of evil'" and must take the fundamentalist regime off the State Department's "terrorism list."

Before analyzing the perils and costs of the grand bargain, it is necessary to discuss the wider political situation and the policy debates within both the American and Iranian sides. I begin with the Iranian side (both opposition and supporters), then proceed with the American side, and finally present my analysis of the grand bargain.

On the Iranian Side: Who's Who Among Iranian Opposition Groups

Opposition groups to the Islamic Republic can be divided into five categories: (1) democratic republicans, (2) monarchists, (3) the People's Mojahedin Organization of Iran, (4) Communists, and (5) ethnic parties (Figure 1).

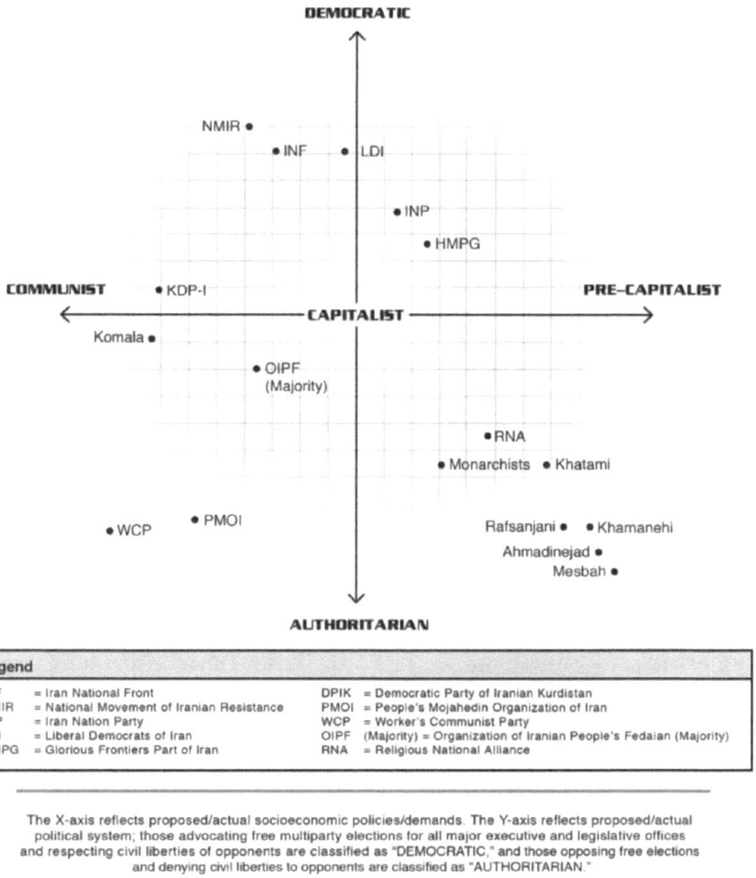

Figure 1. Ideologies of political parties and politicians in Iran, 2007.

Democratic Republicans

The democratic republican groups want to replace the system of clerical rule (*Nezam Velayat Faqih*) with sovereignty of the people, that is, democracy.[6] They advocate civil liberties, pluralist democracy, rule of law, separation of religion and the state, a republican form of government, and free and fair elections. They argue that all citizens should have equal political rights and thus oppose special privileges for any strata (Shiite clerics) and individuals or families (monarchy). They can be divided into two broad categories: established democrats and young democrats.

The established democrats trace their roots to the 1905 Constitutional Revolution and the 1950s oil nationalization movement under Dr. Mossadegh. The most prominent include Iran National Front (*Jebhe Melli Iran*), National Movement of Iranian Resistance (NMIR), Iran Nation party (*Hezb Mellat Iran*), and Liberal Democrats of Iran.[7] The oldest and arguably the largest prodemocracy group operating inside Iran is the Iran National Front (INF), which also operates abroad. The INF was founded in 1949 and led by Mossadegh as prime minister between April 1951 and August 1953, when a CIA-engineered coup overthrew his cabinet. After the 1979 revolution, about one-third of cabinet posts—including foreign minister, defense minister, labor minister, and minister of treasury—were held by INF members. On April 15, 1979, Dr. Karim Sanjabi, INF leader and foreign minister, along with other INF ministers, resigned in protest against arbitrary arrests, gross violations of due process in revolutionary courts, and mass executions by revolutionary courts operating outside the provisional government's authority and under the direct control of Ayatollah Khomeini.[8]

In June 1981 INF was declared apostate by Khomeini and consequently was severely repressed. Between 1997 and 2005, the regime reduced its repression of the activities of the INF, although officially the INF remained illegal and under constant surveillance, harassment, and intimidation, including several hit-and-run attacks. The INF advocates a gradual, step-by-step transition from the incumbent clerical dictatorship to democracy. Issuing communiqués and pronouncements has become the hallmark of the INF. Members of the INF are secular liberal democrats and secular social democrats.

National Movement of Iranian Resistance (NMIR) was led by Dr. Shahpour Bakhtiar, the second highest official of INF. An old nemesis of the shah, Bakhtiar agreed to assume the prime ministership 37 days before the collapse of the monarchy in order to prevent Khomeini's rise to power. Bakhtiar formed NMIR shortly after the revolution. Bakhtiar was assassinated in Paris by agents of the fundamentalist regime on August 6, 1991. Earlier, on April 18, 1991, his deputy, Dr. Abdorrahamn Boroumand, was assassinated in Paris by agents of the fundamentalist regime.[9] By and large NMIR members have been social democrats and secular. They have also tended to be more active and action oriented than INF members. In 2007 many members of NMIR, including its third and fourth highest ranked officials (Dr. Homayoun Mehmaneche and Dr. Ali Shakeri Zand), joined the Iran National Front-Abroad.[10]

The Iran Nation Party (INP) split from the INF in April 1979 when INP members decided to remain in the provisional government's cabinet. The entire cabinet resigned on November 4, 1979, in protest against the fundamentalist takeover of the American embassy in Tehran. In June 1981, after fundamentalists purged President Bani Sadr and captured all levers of power, INP founder and leader, Dariush Forouhar, was imprisoned and severely tortured. In November 1998, "rogue" agents of the Ministry of Intelligence assassinated Dariush Forouhar and his wife, Parvaneh Eskandari-Forouhar, the eminent feminist, prodemocracy activist, prolific poet, and university lecturer. It is widely believed that the official behind the operation was Hojatolislam Mustafa Pour-Mohammadi who became minister of interior in President Mahmoud Ahmadinejad's cabinet in 2005.[11]

There is an emerging category of young democrats who are in their 20s and 30s. The most famous and said to be the most representative is Ahmad Batebi. Other leaders in this category are Manuchehr Mohammadi, the late Akbar Mohammadi (who died in prison in July 2006 after enduring a combination of severe torture, hunger strike, and lack of medical attention), Ali Afshari, and Akbar Atri. Impatient with the gradualism and cautiousness of the INF leadership, the young democrats tend to engage in actions such as civil disobedience and rallies instead of merely issuing endless communiqués. Compared to the established democrats, the young democrats tend to be more action oriented, more hostile to the regime, less hostile to monarchists, and friendlier toward the United States.

The prodemocracy student uprising of July 1999 was organized by this group. They have embraced Mossadegh as the symbol of their desire for a secular democratic republic. Several student organizations have grown inside Iran, but by and large, as a result of repression, they have not been able to organize themselves into strong organizations. Despite severe torture and an initial sentence of execution, Ahmad Batebi has continued his resistance to the regime. He has emerged as the iconic leader of the young democrats. Two organizations that have been formed by members of this category and express the sentiments of some but not all of the members of this category are the Alliance of Iranian Students and Glorious Frontiers party of Iran (HMPG).[12] Both of these organizations had to go into exile after the July 1999 uprising.

In addition to the aforementioned categories, there are large number of individuals and intellectuals, both inside Iran and abroad, who are not members of any organization but are democratic republicans. They usually sign open letters and petitions on various issues such as human rights violations. There are also civil society organizations, both inside and outside Iran, such as human rights organizations, labor syndicates, and women's groups that may be classified as democratic republicans. One of the most interesting developments has been the gradual transformation of *Daftar Tahkim Vahdat* (Office for Fostering Unity), the official umbrella fundamentalist student organization created in 1979 as a federation of various fundamentalist students at universities to counter antifundamentalists students and faculty. Today the majority of *Daftar Tahkim Vahdat* (DTV) members have embraced democracy.[13] In an unusually brave action, its members heckled President Ahmadinejad and burned his portrait when he delivered a speech at Polytechnic University in Tehran on December 11, 2006.[14] One student held a sign stating "Fascist President, Polytechnic is not your place."[15] Several dozen leaders of the DTV have since been imprisoned and beaten. In July 2007, in order to prevent celebrations of the July 1999 uprising, more officials of DTV were imprisoned and beaten.[16]

Monarchists

Iranian monarchists are supporters of the Pahlavi dynasty and want to restore Reza Pahlavi, the son of Mohammad Reza Shah Pahlavi, to the throne.[17] Monarchists are divided into constitutional monarchists and absolute monarchists. Both subcategories condemn the 1979 revolution. The constitutional monarchists state that they want to have freely elected parliamentary democracy with Reza Pahlavi as a constitutional monarch. The main group in this category is the Constitutionalist party of Iran.[18] Reza Pahlavi has repeatedly stated that he embraces this position. The absolutist monarchists support the reestablishment of dictatorship.

People's Mojahedin Organization of Iran

People's Mojahedin Organization of Iran (PMOI), also known as the MKO (Mojahedin Khalq Organization) or MeK (Mojahedin e Khalq), or NCRI (National Council of Resistence of Iran), is led by Masoud Rajavi and his wife, Ms. Maryam Azadanlou-Rajavi.[19] The PMOI was established in 1965 as the result of a split from the Liberation Movement of Iran, which itself had split from the INF in 1961. The PMOI's ideology, "Classless Divine Society," combined a Maoist socioeconomic and political system with an egalitarian interpretation of Islam. In 1972, Masoud Rajavi described the PMOI's notion of freedom as that existing at that time in the Soviet Union and China. According to the U.S. State Department and many other sources, the PMOI assassinated several Americans in Iran in the early 1970s, although in the 1980s the PMOI denied this in order to gain U.S. support for its struggle against the fundamentalist regime.

The PMOI has been and remains highly disciplined and very well organized, although it is today only a fraction of what it was in the early 1980s. In the 1979–1982 period, the PMOI grew to become a large, mass-based movement. In June 1981 the PMOI called for armed struggle against the regime after Khomeini's removal of President Bani Sadr. The armed uprising failed to topple the regime. Rajavi and Bani Sadr went into exile in France. In 1986 the PMOI's headquarters moved to Iraq. The organization became closely allied with Saddam Hussein thereafter. By 1986 the PMOI had been transformed from a leftist guerrilla organization into a terribly dictatorial cult.[20] The PMOI has carried out assassinations of the regime's military, intelligence, and political officials, as well as numerous mortar attacks on the regime's military targets.

In 1997 the U.S. State Department included the PMOI on its foreign terrorist organizations list. The British and the EU soon followed and added the PMOI to their terrorist lists. It is widely argued that the reason PMOI was declared a terrorist organization was to reward the newly elected President Mohammad Khatami for his moderation. The PMOI has been lobbying and litigating to have the terrorism label removed. About 4,000 PMOI fighters in Iraq were disarmed by American forces after the invasion of Iraq and remain under American protection in their camp. The PMOI also has about 5,000 highly committed supporters in Europe.

Communist Groups

Iranian communists are dispersed among more than two dozen organizations. The largest Communist organization in the 1980–1991 period, the Organization of Iranian People's Fedaian (Majority), has ceased to be Communist.[21] Smaller groups remain committed to Marxism-Leninism. Today the most active Communist groups are the Workers' Communist party and the Union of People's Fedaian of Iran.[22] Iranian Communists were very strong on university campuses in the 1970s and 1980s. Today Communists are very weak because of a variety of reasons, including their strong ideological support for a dictatorial form of government. Today's students and intellectuals crave freedom of thought, expression, and elections—all lacunae in Leninism that have undermined the appeal of communism among university students and intellectuals.

Ethnic Parties

Many ethnic communities in Iran feel oppressed by the fundamentalist regime. They include Azerbaijanis, Kurds, Balochis, Arabs, and Turkomen. The regime's *de jure* and *de facto* discrimination against Sunnis (i.e., all Balochis and Turkomen and about half of

Kurds and Arabs), which has gone so far as to destroy Sunni mosques in Mashhad and prevent the construction of even a single Sunni mosque in Tehran, has made these minorities especially enraged at the regime. Increased violence in Balochistan, Khuzestan, Kurdestan, Kermanshahan, and Azerbaijan provinces has occurred in recent years.

The oldest and most powerful ethnic party in Iran is the Democratic party of Iranian Kurdistan (DPIK).[23] The DPIK was a typical pro-Moscow Communist party before the 1979 revolution. However, under the able leadership of Dr. Abdo-Rahman Qassemlou, the DPIK became independent of Moscow, embraced democratic socialism, and became affiliated with the social democratic organization "Socialist International." It also moved away from separatist demands and called for autonomy within a federal Iran. The agents of the Iranian government assassinated Dr. Qassemlou and two of his lieutenants in Vienna on July 13, 1989. His successor, Dr. Sadegh Sharafkandi, along with his two lieutenants and another democratic socialist Iranian, were assassinated in Berlin on September 17, 1992, by agents of the Iranian government (and three members of the Lebanese Hezbollah).[24]

Neither Qassemlou nor subsequent leaders of the DPIK made clear exactly what they meant by autonomy and federalism. The DPIK usually uses the term "federalism based on nationality" [*federalism bar asas meliyat*]. The DPIK refuses to use the term "ethnicity" [*ghomiyat*] to refer to Kurds and other minority groups in Iran (e.g., Azerbaijanis, Turkomen, Arabs, Balochis) and instead uses the term nationality [*meliyat*]. Such usage has led many to believe that by "federalism" the DPIK really means "confederalism" where sovereignty resides in an ethnically demarcated unit. Some statements seem to suggest that the DPIK regards the Kurds in Iran as primarily Iranians, whereas other statements seem to suggest that they are primarily part of the Kurdish nation spread in Iran, Iraq, Turkey, and Syria. Many believe that the ultimate goal of the DPIK is the creation of one Kurdish nation-state joining all Kurds (in Iran, Iraq, Turkey, and Syria) in one state. Reading between the lines, it appears that there is a debate among the DPIK on exactly what their ultimate goal should be.

The leadership and cadres of DPIK operate both inside Iran as well as in Iraqi Kurdistan. In the past seven or eight years, the DPIK has become very close to the United States. In an unprecedented move by any Iranian party, the DPIK congratulated President Bush on his reelection in November 2004. The DPIK can count on the support of several million Kurds in Iran as well as many thousands of guerrillas in Iran and in the Kurdish regions of Iraq.

The second most powerful ethnic party in Iran is the Komala, a Kurdish group.[25] Komala used to be a radical Marxist–Leninist party, but it moved away from communism several years ago. It engages in armed conflict with the regime's coercive apparatuses in the Iranian Kurdish region. In the past five to seven years, Komala, like DPIK, has developed a more positive view of the U.S. role in the region. Komala has several thousand guerrillas who operate in the border Kurdish region of Iran and Iraq. In the past few years, Komala and DPIK were able to resolve their earlier differences and have begun to work and coordinate closely.

In 2006 a small Kurdish group (PJAK) surfaced. It has been allied with the PKK, the radical militant Kurdish party in Turkey. The regime's elite Islamic Revolutionary Guards Corps has exchanged fire with PJAK on numerous occasions.

Several Baloch groups compete among themselves and the central government. The Balochistan United Front of Iran (Republican Federal), Balochistan Peoples party, and Balochistan National Movement – Iran support a republican federal system. Like the statements of DPIK, their statements on "federalism" are vague, and it is not clear whether they mean a federal system like that of the

United States or a confederal system. One group led by Amanoullah Khan Riggi has been accused by other Baloch groups of being monarchist.

The Jondollah Organization of Iran carried out military operations against the regime in early 2007. The regime accused it of being allied with Al Qaeda, but the group immediately denied and condemned the accusation. The organization has stated that it supports a democratic, federal, and secular system in Iran. It is imperative to seek information directly from the various opposition groups themselves because the fundamentalist regime has used proxies to spread false information on opposition groups. The most egregious example may be the regime accusation that Jondollah, a Sunni Baloch group, is Wahhabi and is connected to Al Qaeda. To counter the regime's propaganda, the group changed its name to *Jonbeshe Moghavemat Mardomi Iran* (Peoples Resistance Movement of Iran).[26]

Policies of Iranian Opposition Groups

All opposition groups, including social democrats, liberal democrats, Marxists, monarchists, and ethnic minority parties, have been pursuing regime change. Although they have not succeeded in toppling the fundamentalists, they have delegitimized the regime. Today the regime has lost its ideological hegemony and political legitimacy but not its ability to coerce and subdue. This political bankruptcy stems, in large part, from the resistance of the opposition groups and populace to the regime.

The opposition groups regard the fundamentalist regime to be among the most repressive, brutal, reactionary, and misogynist regimes in the world. Many have categorized it as a form of fascism. A few months after the revolution, Ali Asghar Hajj Sayyed Javadi published a series of newspaper articles criticizing the new system as fascistic. These articles were soon published as a pamphlet titled *Az sedaye paye Fashism ta ghoole Fashism ke dar hale tassalot bar sarasar-e Iran ast* [From Early Steps of Fascism to the Specter of Fascism That Is in the Process of Taking Over All of Iran].[27] Hajj Seyyed Javadi was one of Iran's most respected and courageous intellectuals and Iran's most prominent social democrat who had played a prominent role in the anti-shah revolution. Soon he had to go underground and then into exile when the fundamentalist forces were able to crush liberal and leftist forces that had participated in the revolution.

As early as May 1979, the INF leaders condemned the fundamentalist regime as reactionary and fascistic. In the words of Dr. Sanjabi, the number one leader of the INF:

> We believe that a monopolizing and reactionary force is taking shape in this country. This force cannot ignore and deny Iran's past history. It cannot negate Mossadeq or the significance of the oil nationalization movement. It cannot ignore the importance of pluralism and the freedom of the press. Accusations and intimidations are the manifestations of this fascist and reactionary tendency. The National Front of Iran has the responsibility of resisting reaction and dictatorship.[28]

When it was announced that the Assembly of Experts had written a constitution giving Shiite clerics monopolistic powers, the INF issued a strongly worded 10-page analysis. The document repeatedly calls the system religious dictatorship and repeats the earlier warning about emerging "fascism." The document states:

> Individual and social liberties and rights that have been the goals of the revolution have to be respected in practice. Today, all of these liberties

> are in serious threats, and our country is being taken towards a form of fascism. The offices of political parties and societies have been attacked and shot down. Such meetings have also been attacked and closed down. Safety and security of political and social activities of other groups have been eliminated.[29]

Today most opposition groups regard the regime as fascist or fascistic. The Liberal Democrats of Iran regards the fundamentalist regime as fascist.[30] The Green party of Iran calls the regime religious fascism.[31] The Workers Communist party of Iran also calls the regime fascist.[32] Amir Taheri, a prolific conservative commentator in the Iranian media and a frequent contributor to this journal, has described the regime as fascist.[33] Even Mohsen Sazegara, a former fundamentalist, a founder of the Islamic Revolutionary Guards Corps (IRGC), and the man who wrote the constitution of the IRGC, has used the term "fascist" to describe the system created by the Supreme Leader Ali Khamanehi.[34] Akbar Ganji, another former fundamentalist and current dissident, regards the hard-line faction as fascist.[35] Most interesting, even former President Mohammad Khatami recently referred to some of the hard-line fundamentalists who have been criticizing him as fascist.[36]

Describing Islamic fundamentalism as fascist or fascistic or a form of fascism is not limited to political actors in Iran. Many scholars have also described the system created by Khomeini in the same way.[37] Like fascism, Islamic fundamentalist ideology is explicitly corporatist and organic (i.e., society is conceived of as an organic body in which all of the parts have to cooperate in order to ensure the healthy functioning of the system). Such a political system regards its leader as the brain of the polity that has the right to order others and others have to obey. This form of corporatist ideology explicitly denies civil liberties and the right of dissent. Thus individuals are crushed for the sake of the Islamic state. Like fascism, Islamic fundamentalism attempts to create a cult of personality of its leader.

Islam enjoys a rich tradition that includes both mercifulness and peace as well as violence and aggressive war. Moderate and liberal Muslims regard the merciful and peaceful aspects of Islam to constitute Islam's primary message and soul, whereas violence is interpreted as exceptional and historical. Islamic fundamentalists, on the contrary, regard jihad and violence to be primary aspects of Islam, whereas peace and mercifulness are interpreted as minor aspects practiced only after infidels have been vanquished and dominated.

Islamic fundamentalists excel in manipulating prejudices (usually against religious and ethnic minorities) and xenophobic fears of the masses. Islamic fundamentalists have succeeded in mobilizing the masses not through appealing to their best and most noble desires (e.g., tolerance, coexistence, amity, compassion, mercy) but rather to their basest (e.g., hate, prejudice, revenge, envy) feelings.

Like fascism, Islamic fundamentalism views political violence not as a necessary evil but as a desirable tool to subjugate and intimidate domestic and foreign opponents. Religious rituals and liturgy have been manipulated to create a cult of violence that glamorizes violence. Like fascists, Islamic fundamentalists violently attack ethnic and religious minorities, feminists, liberals, leftists, labor unions, professional associations, and homosexuals. Like European fascists, Islamic fundamentalists tend to pursue an extremely bellicose foreign policy.

Iranian opposition groups (prodemocracy, monarchists, PMOI, Communists, and ethnic parties) oppose appeasement of the regime in general and a grand bargain in particular. For Iranian prodemocracy forces, appeasement of such a brutal dictatorship is immoral and unethical on idealist grounds and counterproductive, on realist grounds.[38] The opposition groups have not criticized the Bush administration for calling the regime evil. For Iranian opposition groups, calling the fundamentalist regime evil is like calling a spade a spade.

Some in the opposition support imposing sanctions on the fundamentalist regime similar to the sanctions imposed on the apartheid regime in South Africa. The Iranian state, under both monarchy and the fundamentalist regime, is a "rentier state," which means that it is highly dependent on oil. As long as oil income flows into the coffers of the state, the ruling regime enjoys a great deal of autonomy from domestic social classes and domestic pressures. If the oil income is stopped, however, the regime could face serious difficulties remaining in power.[39] One of the main reasons that the shah was forced to leave power was the successful strike by workers in the oil fields and oil refineries. Because repression is far more severe under the current regime, which executed several thousands in a matter of weeks (e.g., June–December 1981 and September 1988), a level of repression that simply was not in existence under the monarchy, oil workers cannot be asked to go on strike under a regime that has no reservations about executing thousands of them and thus breaking the strike. Because the oil income cannot be stopped at the point of production, it is necessary to stop it at the point of exchange.

According to the Islamic Republic's Central Bank, oil accounts for about 80 percent of foreign earnings, about 60 percent of government revenues, and about 30 percent of GDP.[40] The government received $55 billion from the export of oil and natural gas in the 2005–2006 fiscal year in comparison to $23 billion in the 2002–2003 fiscal year.[41] All of this income goes directly into the hands of the fundamentalist regime. It is this income that allows the fundamentalists to pay for their coercive apparatuses, provide subsidies to maintain the allegiance of their social base, coopt nonfundamentalists through financial largesse, and prevent the economy from collapsing. By purchasing oil and natural gas from the fundamentalist regime, the outside world is helping it to remain in power. In other words, by purchasing oil and natural gas from the regime, the outside world is producing an impact on the internal struggles in Iran. In effect it conduces to the benefit of the fundamentalists and to the detriment of the opposition. Economic sanctions would deprive the fundamentalists of billions of dollars and thus weaken them substantially. This would in effect enable and empower the Iranian people themselves to undermine the fundamentalist regime. The recent riots after the price of gasoline was raised from about 40 cents a gallon to 50 cents are indications of popular discontent with the economic situation.

Some opposition groups advocate close cooperation with the United States, whereas others have taken a neutral position. The monarchists, DPIK, Komala, and PMOI have welcomed the Bush administration's strong stand against the fundamentalist regime. The PMOI, in particular, has lobbied hard and openly to be taken off the terrorism list. Several prominent groups in the United States have advocated that the United States unleash the PMOI to fight the fundamentalist regime.[42] The most articulate think tank that has taken this position consistently is the Iran Policy Committee headed by the former senior member of the National Security Council staff during President Reagan's administration and several prominent national security experts.[43] The Iran Policy Committee has argued that the United States should expunge the name of the PMOI from the terrorism list and provide it with support so that it can overthrow the regime.[44]

Weaknesses of Opposition to the Regime

Although any of the main opposition groups (democrats, monarchists, PMOI) could conceivably provide a political system and leaders far superior to the incumbent regime, a variety of factors have prevented the success of the opposition. One of the main characteristics of Iranian political culture is excessive self-centeredness. Another characteristic is the inability to cooperate with others for the greater good, punctuated by total obedience to a leader.

All indications are that if there were free and democratic elections, the democratic republicans would win. However, the democratic forces lack a strong party and a charismatic leader to unite and organize the various parties and their social base. Their nonviolent method of struggle has proved to be incapable of convincing a tyrannical and violent oligarchy to accept free elections. Although many in their social base would gladly vote for the democratic forces, they believe that such methods would not succeed and are not willing to sacrifice their jobs, wealth, liberties, and lives in a futile and idealistic struggle against the violent fundamentalists. The personal ambition for power shown by too many individuals, each one believing that all others have to follow his or her leadership, has further dispersed and weakened the democratic forces.

The monarchists have one leader, which is an advantage in Iranian political culture. Monarchy, by its very nature, however, demands special and permanent powers for one person and family (who inherits those powers without periodic elections). Monarchy has provoked intense and irreconcilable opposition from all other opposition groups in Iran. The monarchists' social base is too small to overthrow the regime by itself. Reza Pahlavi has failed to build any coalition. The intense hostilities between democratic republicans and monarchists have prevented any alliance between the two. Monarchists blame the democratic forces for cooperating with Khomeini and overthrowing them, whereas the democrats blame the monarchists for their dictatorship and repression. Moreover, democrats fear that monarchists wish to reimpose their dictatorship and simply do not believe Reza Pahlavi's repeated pledges to respect the vote of the people. Great amounts of time and energy have been spent by republicans and monarchists in debating and attacking one another instead of concentrating their activities on the fundamentalist regime. It appears that the only way to generate trust would be for Reza Pahlavi to renounce the monarchy and mobilize his supporters into a conservative republican party. Only such a creative and courageous move would unequivocally prove his commitment to democracy and virtually guarantee a broad based coalition capable of mobilizing the masses and undermining the fundamentalist regime.

The PMOI is by far the most organized and disciplined group in Iran. It is capable of carrying out military operations inside Iran and mobilizing many thousands of its supporters abroad. Because of its ideology, history, and leadership, it is resented and feared by the vast majority of Iranians. It is clear that PMOI neither could win any major election nor overthrow the regime. It is also clear, however, that it has enough muscle, organization, and committed members to be a significant player in Iranian politics. Its dictatorial leadership has alienated it from all of the major opposition groups.

Ethnic minority parties have proved that they are able to cause a great many problems for the regime, but they have not succeeded in making alliances with national parties. If a formula could be found that would both safeguard the civil rights of ethnic minorities and preserve the territorial integrity of Iran, a broad coalition would be possible. As long as ethnic parties demand "autonomy," it will be virtually impossible for national opposition parties to make coalitions with them.

In addition to the aforementiond factors, a number of cleavages exist among as well as within opposition groups and the society at large. Such opposition groups

- engage in armed struggle or nonviolent methods of struggle or a combination of the two;

- advocate the establishment of a unitary system or an American-style federal system or a confederacy based on ethno-sectarian autonomy;
- advocate economic sanctions or oppose them or remain silent;
- cooperate with the United States or remain neutral in the confrontation between the United States and the fundamentalist regime;
- enter into overt or covert relations with the United States;
- call on the people to vote for reformist members of the fundamentalist oligarchy under certain circumstances or advocate a boycott of elections.

These cleavages have led many opposition elements to spend a great deal of time debating and attacking other opposition elements instead of attacking the fundamentalist regime. The primary beneficiary has been the regime.

In sum, although the vast majority of the Iranian public opposes the fundamentalist regime and strong opposition groups exist, several serious issues divide the opposition groups. The failure of one leader (or a handful of leaders cooperating with one another) to emerge and present a formula capable of uniting the opposition has prevented the widespread dissatisfaction with the regime from coalescing and coming to fruition. This kind of divisiveness has enabled the regime to contain and suppress numerous actions by students, women, workers, writers, journalists, urban poor, human rights activists, and minorities.

On the Iranian Side: The Fundamentalist Regime

Great amounts of ink, paper, and byte have been devoted to analyzing the regime. Thus only a few sentences will be added to this subject here. All fundamentalist officials—hardline and reformist alike—strongly resent President Bush's description of the regime as part of the "axis of evil." Limited, issue-based dialogue has been conducted numerous times between regime officials and the United States. Former Presidents Mohammad Khatami and Ali Akbar Rafsanjani and their supporters have advocated a grand bargain. President Mahmoud Ahmadinejad and his followers are thought to be pushing for war.[45] The Supreme Leader Ali Khamanehi has taken different positions at various times depending on the circumstances.

On the American Side

In an excellent article Kurt Campbell and Derek Chollet have described various foreign policy "cliques" in the post–September 11 period without mentioning their policy proposals toward Iran.[46] In this section the policies of some of these groups will be discussed in order to provide the context within which to elucidate the grand bargain proposed by Leverett and Mann.

American neoconservatives and liberal hawks advocate regime change.[47] For the neoconservatives and liberal hawks, the fundamentalist regime is truly evil and bent on undermining pro-Western governments in the region and can be toppled. Specific policies proposed include providing moral and political support to the opposition; providing financial and political assistance to opposition groups; imposing economic sanctions; sabotaging nuclear facilities; carrying out surgical strikes at nuclear facilities; conducting massive military strikes at coercive apparatuses; unleashing full-scale invasion; or a combination thereof.[48]

Rapprochement with the Fundamentalist Regime

Several groups promote rapprochement with the regime. Some are realists, whereas others are idealists. The most influential include "Oldsmobile Conservatives" in the Republican party and "Globalists" in the Democratic party.[49] James Kurth has referred to the perspectives of Oldsmobile Conservatives as "conservative/realist."[50] This group includes prominent Republicans such as General Brent Scowcroft (national security adviser to President George H. W. Bush), Richard Armitage (deputy secretary of state under President George W. Bush), and Richard Haass (director of the State Department's Policy Planning Staff from 2001 to 2003 and president of the Council on Foreign Relations since 2003). Prominent Democrats are increasingly promoting a similar position. *The National Interest* has emerged as the main journal that publishes the views of prorapprochement realists.

The most detailed and sophisticated policy proposals promoting rapprochement with the fundamentalist regime are advocated by Ray Takeyh, Anatol Lieven, John Hulsman, and Gary Sick.[51] Dr. Ray Takeyh was a professor at the National War College and the National Defense University. He is currently a senior fellow at the Council on Foreign Relations and a contributing editor to *The National Interest*. Dr. Anatol Lieven is a senior research fellow at the New America Foundation, a contributing editor to *The National Interest*, and a former senior associate at the Carnegie Endowment for International Peace. Dr. John Hulsman was a senior research fellow at the Heritage Foundation. He is currently a contributing editor to *The National Interest* and a scholar in residence at the Alfred von Oppenheim Center for European Studies in Berlin, Germany. Dr. Gary Sick served on the National Security Council under Presidents Ford, Carter, and Reagan. He is currently affiliated with Columbia University's School of International and Public Affairs as adjunct professor and a senior research scholar.

Their argument is based on the following beliefs: (1) the fundamentalist regime is here to stay for the foreseeable future; (2) the United States simply is unable to invade and overthrow the regime; (3) mere military strikes on nuclear installations would provoke retaliation on the United States and its allies with grave economic, strategic, and political consequences that they could not absorb; and (4) the regime can be convinced to play by the norms of international conduct by a combination of carrots and sticks. The last belief is based on the assumption that the rationality that worked with Communists (which formed the foundation for containment, deterrence, and mutual assured destruction [MAD]) will also work with Islamic fundamentalists. They dismiss the fundamentalist ideological principles of mass martyrdom (e.g., guaranteed entrance to paradise) and rapture as determinants of the foreign policy of the fundamentalist regime.

For the realists in this group, interests, not ideology (communist or Islamic fundamentalist), play the main role in the making of foreign policy. For them, stability is the primary if not the sole concern. Issues such as democracy, human rights, and forms of government should be ignored for the sake of stability. For the realists in this group, dialogue, detente, and rapprochement do not constitute appeasement. For them, American power is very limited, as has been made painfully clear by the war in Iraq.

For the idealists in this group, the main fear is that President Bush will take America to yet another war in the Middle East based on a false pretext or exaggerated evidence and before all diplomatic avenues have been exhausted. Some are willing to accept the possession of nuclear weapons by the fundamentalist regime.[52] Globalist democrats are not against the use of force; nor do they maintain that issues of human rights are irrelevant. After all, many in the Clinton administration did use force on many occasions, including massive force in Haiti, Bosnia, and Kosovo and surgical strikes in Iraq and Afghanistan.

Antiappeasement Realists

This group includes prominent Republicans and Democrats such as Senator John McCain (R.–Arizona) and R. James Woolsey (director of the CIA under President Clinton). The most detailed and sophisticated policy proposals by antiappeasement realists were articulated by the late Fereydoun Hoveyda, James Kurth, and Peter Brookes.[53] A frequent contributor to this journal, Ambassador Hoveyda was prerevolution Iran's ambassador to the United Nations. Dr. Kurth is the editor of *Orbis*. Dr. Brookes is senior fellow at the Heritage Foundation. Brookes served as the deputy assistant defense secretary in the George W. Bush administration, in the CIA's Directorate of Operations, and in the State Department.

The most prestigious scholarly and policy oriented journals that publish the analyses of antiappeasement realists include *American Foreign Policy Interests* and *Orbis*. It is imperative to add that both of these journals publish analyses of various realist traditions. Think tanks that include analysts that could be classified as antiappeasement realists include the National Committee on American Foreign Policy (NCAFP), Foreign Policy Research Institute (FPRI), the Heritage Foundation, and the Washington Institute for Near East Policy (WINEP).[54]

This group of realists views the fundamentalist regime in Iran as a serious threat to the United States. Some in this group argue that talking with one's enemy is necessary. Diplomacy is part of containment that was carried out with the former Soviet Union. Diplomacy, for example, has borne fruit in confrontations with North Korea and Libya. As a matter of principle, all realists, including antiappeasement realists, advocate diplomacy as a tool that should always be on the table. What distinguishes this group of realists is that they advocate that the United States should neither give in to the illegitimate demands of the fundamentalist regime nor be perceived as though it were willing to appease the regime. Unlike liberal hawks and neoconservatives, who oppose holding talks with a regime so odious that one ought to be trying to overthrow it, antiappeasement realists do not oppose talks and diplomacy with Iran.

Some in this group argue that dialogue with a hostile regime should be entered into only after a careful cost-benefit analysis. Put another way, engagement could be worse than containment or rollback. According to David Rivkin, American engagement with the Iranian regime would bestow legitimacy on the regime and would undermine the multilateral sanctions at the United Nations Security Council.[55]

The problem with the particular case of Iran has been compounded by the oligarchic nature of the regime's rift with factions and individuals, not one of whom seems to be able to speak with authority for long periods of time. In other words, the obstacle to talks with Iran has had more to do with Iran's lack of a leader with authorization to carry out talks with the United States than with its slogan of "Death to America" or its policies of assisting those who have carried out terrorist acts against Americans. One day Supreme Leader Ali Khamanehi condemns any one who proposes talking with "the Great Satan" as a traitor or a person of dishonor, a few days later he allows a person to carry out such discussions, and a few days or weeks later he dismisses the official who had engaged in the talks.

The perceptions of the antiappeasement realists about the wisdom of holding talks with the fundamentalist regime can be plotted along a continuum. At one end of the spectrum, Woolsey, Brookes, and the Heritage Foundation oppose holding talks with the fundamentalist regime. In their view, under current circumstances, such talks would be more harmful than beneficial. At the other end, the NCAFP is willing to consider talks if an official with authority were available to undertake that responsibility. Hoveyda was located in between, as is Kurth.

These realists view the fundamentalist regime as essentially an expansionist power and regard concessions made to it as appeasement. They argue that the actual policies of the regime since coming to power have repeatedly shown its determination to undermine pro-Western governments and install violent extremist, anti-American proxies and clients in Iraq, Lebanon, Bahrain, Afghanistan, Saudi Arabia, and Palestine. Moreover, they argue, the regime is committed to the destruction of Israel.

The realists have a point. Iran's export of the fundamentalist Islamic revolution to the entire world via violent jihad is a constitutional mandate. The constitution created by the fundamentalists in 1979 states:

> With due attention to the Islamic content of the Iranian Revolution, the Constitution provides the necessary basis for ensuring the continuation of the Revolution at home and abroad. In particular, in the development of international relations, the Constitution will strive with other Islamic and popular movements to prepare the way for the formation of a single world community (in accordance with the Koranic verse "This your community is a single community, and I am your Lord, so worship Me" [21:92]), and to assure the continuation of the struggle for the liberation of all deprived and oppressed peoples in the world....
>
> An Ideological Army
>
> In the formation and equipping of the country's defense forces, due attention must be paid to faith and ideology as the basic criteria. Accordingly, the Army of the Islamic Republic of Iran and the Islamic Revolutionary Guards Corps are to be organized in conformity with this goal, and they will be responsible not only for guarding and preserving the frontiers of the country, but also for fulfilling the ideological mission of jihad in God's way; that is, extending the sovereignty of God's law throughout the world (this is in accordance with the Koranic verse "Prepare against them whatever force you are able to muster, and strings of horses, striking fear into the enemy of God and your enemy, and others besides them." [8:60])[56]

These realists argue that appeasement did not work with Hitler in 1938 and it will not work with fundamentalists today. Any concession would not only further embolden them but would also provide them with additional resources to carry out their expansionism. The interests of the United States and those of the fundamentalists are irreconcilable. Appeasement would allow the fundamentalist regime to choose the time, place, and manner of confrontation. Of most significance, additional time would enhance the fundamentalist regime's capability to acquire nuclear weapons, thus dramatically altering the balance of power in the region and increasing the likelihood that war and nuclear exchange would produce a far more devastating outcome than the stronger early policy. Unlike the Soviet and the Chinese Communists, whose ideology was materialist and rationally bounded and who believed that time was on their side, Islamic fundamentalists combine expansionism with an irrational metaphysical zeal for mass suicide, a combination that will not respond logically to concepts of MAD.[57] In such hands, nuclear weapons would not bring Clausewitzian restraint for the sake of preserving the state[58] but would provide the means for bringing Armageddon and the hoped for Shiite rapture.

This group of realists regards the prorapprochement realists as suffering from a prostatus quo bias. Such a bias has been responsible for overestimating the strength and legitimacy of many regimes and for underestimating the fragility and crises of legitimacy, thereby discounting the likelihood of regime change and rollback as a realistic policy. Antiappeasement realists share with neoconservatives and liberal hawks the belief that it is necessary to oppose appeasement and stand up to expansionist aggressive powers.

Reconfigured Containment

The high costs of regime change (at least in the short term) and the high, long-term costs both of limited issue based dialogue and the grand bargain seem to have given impetus to two new options involving low, short-term costs. One can be called tripartite containment and the other ethnic destabilization. Some postulate that a new strategy is emerging for a tripartite containment of Iran by the United States, Israel, and Sunni Arab states (Saudi Arabia, Egypt, Jordan, and the Gulf Cooperation Council, an organization composed of the littoral Arab states of the Persian Gulf).[59] This policy can be described as containment, although it is more a short- term tactic than a long-term strategy. If in fact the Iranian regime is developing nuclear weapons, such containment would neither change the regime's behavior nor its nature. It may, however, reduce its ability to expand its influence in the region. Such tripartite coordination may be particularly effective in Iraq and Lebanon if augmented by increased forces and resources on the ground.

The least discussed policy option is assistance to ethno-sectarian minorities in Iran. Although the fundamentalist regime discriminates against all Iranians who are not fundamentalist, including those from the majority Persian ethnicity (slightly more than half of the population), non-Persians and non-Shiites feel especially oppressed merely because of their ethnic or religious or ethno-religious backgrounds.[60] Iran's minorities such as Azeris, Kurds (half are Sunni), Balochis (almost all are Sunni), Arabs (half are Sunni), and Turkomen (all are Sunni) live primarily in the sensitive border regions. Some suffer from *de jure* or *de facto* discrimination. Sunni Kurds (unlike Shiite Kurds) exhibit irredentist aspirations that have only increased in recent years.[61] In the past few years, mass demonstrations by Azeris as well as major violent clashes between the regime's coercive apparatuses and the Arabs, Kurds, and Balochis have taken place. The result has been hundreds of deaths on all sides.[62] The policy may be designed to put pressure on the regime in order to frighten it into compromising or to create enough trouble to compel the regime to redirect its forces from expansionism into internal security (containment)[63] or to prepare for an invasion (regime change)[64] in the not too distant future. Thus depending on their ultimate objective, many groups may promote this policy.[65]

Military Strikes

Many have advocated surgical military strikes on the nuclear facilities. If the fundamentalist regime did not retaliate, this tactic would postpone the nuclear program. But if the regime did retaliate, such action would begin a major war. If the regime were able to close off the Strait of Hormuz, it would be able to cut off oil shipments, thus crippling the world economy. There is no reason to believe that merely striking nuclear facilities would serve as a trigger for mass uprisings, as some in Washington seem to hope, the reason being that with coercive apparatuses intact, the regime would not only have the power to crush any uprising but would also have the added motivation and anger to do so. One could only expect a mass uprising if the military strikes target coercive apparatuses such as the Islamic

Revolutionary Guards Corps, the Basij militia, the Ministry of Intelligence, and so on.

Many believe that because of the wars in Iraq and Afghanistan, the United States lacks the capability to make massive military strikes; therefore, the United States has to give in to the fundamentalist regime. Others believe that the Air Force and Navy have remained pretty much intact; therefore, the United States is capable of using massive missile and aerial attacks on the nuclear facilities and coercive apparatuses of the regime. Whether there will be a mass uprising resulting in the overthrow of the regime or, conversely, whether the masses will support the regime cannot be known beforehand. The behavior and public statements of top officials of the United States, the fundamentalist regime, and the opposition groups leading up to military strikes could have a determining effect on the reaction of vast numbers of the Iranian people. There is little doubt that there will be fundamentalists who will put up a fierce fight. There is also little doubt that the United States could arm and unleash a number of groups against the regime.

The belief among many in Washington that there is no military solution has caused many to advocate a grand bargain. The most detailed proposal has been the one advanced by Leverett and Mann.

A Grand Bargain

The Iraq Study Group (ISG), chaired by two prominent statesmen, James Baker and Lee Hamilton, promoted a limited, issue-based dialogue with the leaders of Iran and Syria in order to help the United States exit from Iraq. In their December 22 op-ed article in *The New York Times*, Leverett and Mann took aim at the ISG and argued that the policy of a limited, issue-based dialogue is doomed to failure. It reiterated the proposal of a grand bargain that Leverett had made in a longer study. In the earlier study, Leverett opposed the policy of regime change and harshly criticized the Bush administration for not accepting the May 2003 grand bargain.[66] Leverett articulated a new grand bargain.

Leverett is aware that a grand bargain may be regarded as appeasement by many. In an op-ed article published in the January 24, 2006, edition of *The New York Times*, Leverett wrote: "Moreover, Ahmadinejad's execrable rhetoric about Israel and the Holocaust threatens to make future Western engagement look like appeasement." Then he proceeded to describe his proposal: "Such a framework would . . . offer all parts of the Iranian political spectrum–even the hard-liners around Ahmadinejad—something they want: recognition of Iran's leading regional role."

Leverett and Mann have continued to promote a grand bargain despite the fundamentalist regime's more bellicose policies and rhetoric such as supporting the Lebanese Hezbollah in the summer of 2006 and holding an official conference on the Holocaust on December 11–12, 2006.[67] It is significant that the conference was organized by Mohammad Ali Ramin who is a top adviser to President Ahmadinejad and is the secretary of "*Rayeheh Khosh Khedmat*," the electoral list of supporters of Ahmadinejad for the 2006 elections.[68] In a lecture at the University of Gilan on May 30, 2006, Mr. Ramin said:

> Among the Jews there have always been harmful and wicked elements who killed God's prophets and stood against justice and rights, and this ethnic group has done the most damage to the human society throughout history, and another group among them has engaged in conspiracies, inflicting harm and cruelties on other nations and ethnic groups. . . . There are many accusations against the Jews throughout history, among them that they are the cause of spreading of diseases

such as plague and typhus, because the Jews are very dirty persons.[69]

A Fatal Flaw in Any Grand Bargain

The essential component of their grand bargain (or any grand bargain) is the assumption that the fundamentalist regime will honestly declare all of the sites and the dimensions of its nuclear weapons program. This assumption goes against the actual history and behavior of the regime. The regime kept its nuclear program secret for 18 years until it was disclosed by the PMOI. Far more significant is the fact that the regime explicitly deceived the EU-3 (Britain, France, and Germany).

In the October 2003 meeting among regime officials and the foreign ministers of the EU-3, the regime explicitly agreed to provide full disclosure to the foreign ministers and the International Atomic Energy Agency (IAEA) in exchange for the EU-3's agreement that it would oppose the American policy of referring Iran's case to the UN Security Council. In February 2006, during intense intraelite fighting, Hassan Rouhani revealed that Ahmadinejad and his hard-line colleagues had attacked Rouhani and the previous team as both incompetent and weak and claimed that their policies were responsible for undermining Iran's position in the nuclear conflict. Rouhani responded by publishing his remarks to the High Council of the Islamic Cultural Revolution.[70] Rouhani said that in October 2003, after serious deliberations that included all of the main leaders of the regime, they collectively decided not to reveal all of the secrets to the Europeans and the IAEA because doing so would have caused Iran's file to be referred to the Security Council. One such case was the P2 centrifuge case. The regime was not aware that the Libyan government had disclosed all of its nuclear programs to the United States and Britain. Thus the fundamentalist regime decided not to reveal that it had secretly purchased the highly sophisticated P2 centrifuge plans. Because of the Libyan disclosures, the EU-3 and the IAEA were aware of the person who had sold P2 centrifuge plans to Iran. Rouhani stated that the exposure of Iran's explicit deceptions caused the EU-3 to mistrust Iran.[71] This disclosure led the EU to support the American policy of referring Iran to the Security Council. It is imperative to add that engaging in deception about its nuclear file is not an exception for the Iranian regime. It has a long history of explicit lies such as its public denials of the assassinations of dissidents abroad despite the fact that its agents have been arrested, convicted, and imprisoned in many Western European countries. Although the regime has successfully lobbied for the extradition of the imprisoned assassins to Iran, it denies that those agents were sent by the regime.[72] Lying is allowed in Shiite Islam under the practice of "*taghiyeh*" [lying, deception, dissimulation].

The belief that the regime has not declared all of its nuclear facilities is widespread. It involves the so-called problem of known and unknown nuclear facilities. In Leverett's words: "Numerous analyses have raised serious doubts that U.S. military strikes against Iran's nuclear infrastructure would delay significantly its nuclear development because of profound uncertainty about the reliability and comprehensiveness of target selection, the possibility that 'unknown' facilities are at least as close to producing weapons-grade fissile materials as 'known' facilities." . . .

There is an internal logical inconsistency in Leverett's argument. On the one hand, Leverett uses this belief to argue against military strikes. On the other hand, Leverett's grand bargain is based on the belief that the regime will honestly provide a complete list of its hitherto "unknown" nuclear facilities and programs to the United States and will agree to dismantle them. In addition, the regime has the added incentive to continue to lie rather than to change its pattern of lying. Continuing to keep the "unknown" facilities "unknown" could enable the regime to take advantage of collaboration in the "known" facilities to advance its technological acquisitions in the "unknown" facilities. Once the regime developed nuclear weapons in the "unknown" facilities, it could then suspend the grand bargain.

Fatal Attractions of the Grand Bargain

In addition to the fundamental flaw in any grand bargain, the grand bargain that Leverett proposed in the longer study includes principles that would cause the fundamentalist rulers to reject it. The Leverett grand bargain includes implementing internationally recognized human rights conventions,[73] recognizing Israel via accepting UN Security Council Resolutions 242 and 338, and stopping assistance to Lebanese Hezbollah and Hamas. If the regime were to respect the basic human rights of the Iranian people, it would not last long. The fundamentalist regime needs massive coercion in order to remain in power, a fact obvious to regime officials but one that Leverett fails to take into account. It was one thing for Khatami in 2003 to say that if the Palestinians accept a deal with the Israelis, Iran would not be more Palestinian than the Palestinians; it is quite another for Khamanehi and Ahmadinejad today to accept Security Council resolutions officially recognizing the existence of Israel, a nation they want to wipe off the map. It is imperative to add that even in May 2003, Khamanehi did not accept all of the features of the roadmap.

The roadmap offered by the regime in 2003 reflected the interests of the fundamentalists ruling Iran at that particular moment. But would any grand bargain be in the interests of the United States?

The long-term interests of the United States involve cultivating and maintaining the good will of the Iranian people. The United States was intensely hated in Iran because of the CIA-engineered 1953 coup (which overthrew Iran's democratic government of Dr. Mossadegh) and the support the United States gave to the dictatorial regime of the shah. Since the early 1990s, however, Iranians have been one of the most pro-American populations in the world.

What Do Iranians Think?

Because of the highly repressive and brutal nature of the regime in Iran, one cannot expect respondents to give honest answers to sensitive questions, especially when they might lose their jobs or be imprisoned, tortured, or executed. Thus scientific polling, in which interviewers go from house to house or conduct interviews by telephone, is not a reliable indicator of genuine attitudes. A better indication of public sentiments may be various Internet polls in which the respondents believe that they can express their opinions safely. However, such Internet polls are not scientific and have to be taken with great caution.

In early 2003 a large Internet poll of students of the Amir Kabir University (the second most prestigious university in Iran) was conducted by the *Daftar Tahkim Vahdat*, the official student umbrella group. The result was posted on the university's student Web site until they were ordered to remove it. In the poll only 6 percent of the students said that they supported the hard-liners, whereas 4 percent said they supported the reformists within the regime. A mere 5 percent said they supported the return of the former monarchy. Of most significance, 85 percent of the students said that they would support the establishment of a secular and democratic republic.[74] Although one cannot extrapolate from the sentiments of university students the attitudes of the entire population, one can appreciate the extent of the unpopularity of the fundamentalist regime among important segments of the population.

Based in the United States, Iranian.com is the oldest and one of the most widely read Iranian e-magazines. In one poll respondents indicated that they believed that Iranians are the most pro-American group in the Islamic world.[75]

President George W. Bush is popular among Iranians because he has repeatedly condemned the fundamentalist rulers while praising the Iranian people and their culture and history.[76] This explains why Persian speakers were the only group in an October 2004 BBC World Service online poll that supported Bush over Senator Kerry.[77] The various languages of the respondents were Arabic, English, Spanish, Persian, Russian, Urdu, Hindi, Portuguese, Chinese traditional, and Chinese Simplified. The number of total respondents was 73,547. Whereas 71 percent of all of the respondents voted for Kerry, only 20 percent voted for Bush. Among the 5,492 Persian-speaking respondents, 51 percent voted for Bush, 42 percent voted for Kerry, and 7 percent voted for Nader.

Similar sentiments were evident in another Internet poll at Iranian.com. Although in one poll the respondents in large proportions (54% to 17%) supported the Democratic party over the Republican party,[78] in another poll at the same site respondents supported Bush over Kerry for the 2004 election.[79] Senator Kerry's perceived failure to distinguish between the Iranian people and the ruling regime and his repeated calls for rapprochement with the fundamentalist regime were the main reasons for his lack of support among Iranians, including many Iranian liberals.

These Internet polls vindicate what Thomas Friedman wrote in *The New York Times*. According to Friedman,

> Funny enough, the one country on this side of the ocean that would have elected Mr. Bush is not in Europe, but in the Middle East: it's Iran, where many young people apparently hunger for Mr. Bush to remove their despotic leaders, the way he did in Iraq.
>
> An Oxford student who had just returned from research in Iran told me that young Iranians were "loving anything their government hates," such as Mr. Bush, "and hating anything their government loves." Tehran is festooned in "Down With America" graffiti, the student said, but when he tried to take pictures of it, the Iranian students he was with urged him not to. They said it was just put there by their government and was not how most Iranians felt.
>
> Iran, he said, is the ultimate "red state."[80]

Why have Iranians who had so intensely hated the United States between 1953 and the late 1980s become so staunchly pro-American since the early 1990s? By extension, why is there no such positive sentiment toward other countries that have had friendly relations with the Iranian government? The answer to these questions could help guide American policy toward Iran.

The overwhelming majority of Iranians hated the shah's dictatorship. U.S. support for that dictatorship caused Iranians to hate the United States. Similarly, the overwhelming majority of Iranians have come to hate the fundamentalist regime, whose human rights record is far worse than that of the shah's. Those governments that have friendly relations with the fundamentalist regime are viewed negatively by the Iranian public. The Iranian public has high regard for the United States because the widely held perception is that it has stood by the Iranian people and has opposed the ruling fundamentalist dictatorship while Europeans and Russians have put profits before concerns over human rights and democracy in Iran.

A grand bargain would be in the interests of the United States only if one accepts the assumption that the regime is legitimate in the eyes of the vast majority of the Iranian people. If that assumption is valid, then one would expect that Iranians would continue to hate the United States and have positive feelings toward those who have had friendly political and economic relations with the regime. However, the well-known pro-American sentiment among Iranians casts doubt on that assumption.

The United States has won the hearts and minds of a new generation of Iranians. A grand bargain, which is regarded by vast sectors of the Iranian public as appeasement of their tormentors, would undermine that hard-earned positive sentiment.

About the Author

Masoud Kazemzadeh is associate professor, Department of Political Science, Sam Houston State University.

Notes

1. www.tcf.org/list.asp?type=PB&pubid=595

2. On February 14, 2007, *The Washington Post* placed a copy of the proposal on its Web site: www.washingtonpost.com/wp-srv/world/documents/us_iran_roadmap.pdf

3. The emphases in bold letters and the grammatical errors are in the original. I made only a few corrections to the obvious typos.

4. "MKO" refers to the People's Mojahedin Organization of Iran (PMOI), a militant antifundamentalist organization stationed in Iraq since the mid-1980s. The Iranian government uses the acronym MKO instead of the actual name used by the PMOI.

5. See www.nytimes.com/packages/pdf/opinion/20070429_iran-memo-expurgated.pdf. This document, provided by Iranian officials, includes the more specific demands.

6. Unlike Iranian observers, many Western journalists have confused the terms "reformists" and "democrats" in describing Iranian political actors. In Iran "reformists" refers to those who want to reform the fundamentalist system of clerical rule in order to preserve and prolong it. President Mohammad Khatami is a prime example. "Democrats" refers to those who want to replace the system of clerical rule with democracy. The Council of Guardians, which vets candidates for various offices, has allowed many reformist members of the fundamentalist oligarchy to run. Its duty is to prevent those who oppose that system (e.g., democrats) from running.

7. www.jebhemelli.net/; www.melliun.org/nehzatm.htm; www.melliun.org/hezbemel02.htm; and www.iranliberal.com/

8. Sanjabi was one of Iran's foremost constitutional law experts. He was professor and dean of the Faculty of Law at the University of Tehran, served as the Iranian judge at the International Court of Justice during the Anglo-Iranian Oil Company case, and been minister of education in Mossadegh's cabinet in the 1950s.

9. www.abfiran.org/english/aboutboroumand.php

10. www.melliun.org/jebhehkharej02.htm

11. Human Rights Watch, "Ministers of Murder: Iran's New Security Cabinet" (December 2005), www.hrw.org/backgrounder/mena/iran1205/. In addition to the assassination of INP leaders in the fall of 1998, the regime assassinated Mohammad Mokhtari, Mohammad Jaafar Pouyandeh, and Majid Sharif, all prominent writers, in what became known as the chain murders of intellectuals.

12. http://daneshjooyan.org/; http://marze-porgohar.org/index.php?l=1

13. www.advarnews.us/

14. Frances Harrison, "'Mass Purges' at Iran Universities," BBC (December 20, 2006), http://news.bbc.co.uk/2/hi/middle_east/6196069.stm; www.boston.com/news/world/middleeast/articles/2007/06/22/iranian_dissidents_face_broad_crackdown/

15. Michael Weissenstein, "Iranian Dissidents Face Broad Crackdown," AP, June 22, 2007, www.boston.com/news/world/middleeast/

articles/2007/06/22/iranian_dissidents_face_broad_crackdown/

16. Freedom House, "On the Eighth Anniversary of Violent Attacks against Student Protestors, Iranians Again Face Brutal Repression" (July 10, 2007), www.freedomhouse.org/template.cfm?page = 70&release = 526; Ali Akbar Dareini, "Iranian Police Raid Prodemocracy Group," AP (July 9, 2007), www.guardian.co.uk/worldlatest/story/0,,-6767525,00.html; Golnaz Esfandiari, "Iran: Student Activists Detained on Anniversary of Unrest," Radio Free Europe/Radio Liberty (July 9, 2007), www.rferl.org/featuresarticle/2007/07/1f3d2934-15cd-4666-ad08-c5f71f6538f9.html; "Iran Arrests 16 Students on Student Riots Anniversary" *Middle East Times* (July 10, 2007), www.metimes.com/storyview.php?StoryID = 20070710-063647-7082r

17. www.rezapahlavi.org/index.htm

18. www.irancpi.org/

19. www.ncr-iran.org/

20. Ervand Abrahamian, *The Iranian Mojahedin* (New Haven, 1989).

21. www.fadai.org/

22. The Workers Communist party Web site is www.wpiran.org/, and Union of People's Fedaian of Iran Web site is www.etehadefedaian.org/

23. www.pdki.org/

24. Masoud Kazemzadeh, "God's Assassins: The Lebanese Hezbollah and the Fundamentalist Regime Ruling Iran," www.iranian.com (July 16, 2006), www.iranian.com/Kazemzadeh/2006/July/Hezbollah/index.html

25. www.komala.org/

26. See its Internet site at www.jonbesh-mardom.blogspot.com

27. Ali Asghar Hajj Sayyed Javadi, *Az sedaye paye Fashism ta ghoole Fashism ke darhale tassalot bar sarasar-e Iran ast* [From early steps of Fascism to the specter of Fascism that is in the process of taking over all of Iran] (Tehran: no publisher, no date, reprinted in Berlin, Germany: Koshesh Bararayeh Pishbord Nehzat Melli Iran Publishers, Esfand 1359 [1980]).

28. *Peygham-e Emrouz* (May 31, 1979), translated and cited in Ali Rahnema and Farhad Nomani, *The Secular Miracle: Religion, Politics and Economic Policy in Iran* (London, 1990), 200, 232.

29. Iran National Front, *Nazar Jebhe Melli Iran dar bareh Shoraha va Majles Khobregan: Majles Khobregan bayad dar tasmimat khod betore asasi tajdid nazar konad* [The Perspective of the Iran National Front on the Councils and the Assembly of Experts: The Assembly of Experts Has to Make Fundamental Changes in Its Decisions] Aban 1358 [October 1979].

30. See the analyses of two of the founders and leaders of the Liberal Democrats of Iran: Hassan Behgar, "Jojeh fashistha sar az tokhm dar miavarand!" [Fascist chicks are hatching] (July 3, 2005), www.iranliberal.com/Maghaleh-ha/Hassan_Behgar/jojeh.htm, and Ramin Kamran, "Bohrani ke dar raah ast" [The upcoming crisis], www.iranliberal.com/Maghaleh-ha/Ramin_Kamran/051123_Ahmadi_W_2_RaminK.htm

31. See www.iran-e-sabz.org/statements/Conference.html, and www.iran-e-sabz.org/articles/article5.html

32. See the article by one of its top leaders, Hamid Taqvaee, "Round two of the election puppet show in Iran" (June 22, 2005), www.wpiran.org/English/wb183%20round%20two%20of%20election%20show%20in%20Iran%20HT.htm

33. Amir Taheri, "Fascism in Muslim Countries," *American Foreign Policy Interests*, vol. 26, no. 1 (February 2004): 21–30.

34. Mohsen Sazegara, "Iran's Road to Democracy," *Open Democracy* (2005), www.opendemocracy.net/debates/article-3-128-2413.jsp

35. Akbar Ganji, *Talaqi fashisti az din va hokumat* [The Fascist Interpretation of Religion and Government], (Tehran: Tarh-e No, 2000). In 2000, when he wrote this book, Ganji was still a supporter of the fundamentalist regime. In 2002, Ganji changed his previous position and began to advocate the replacement of the fundamentalist regime and its constitution with democracy.

36. In Khatami's words: "What is bad is, under the name of Islam, to expel those who hold a different taste; this is not Islam, this is fascism." Marjan Towhidi, interview with Mostafa Tajzadeh, titled "Osolgarayan ba bohran karaee va mashrooiyat movajehe shodeand" [Fundamentalists confront a crisis of competency and legitimacy] (July 5, 2007), www.iran-emrooz.net/index.php?/politic2/more/13410 (accessed July 5, 2007), my translation.

37. For a discussion of competing paradigms in the study of Islamic fundamentalism, see Masoud Kazemzadeh, "Teaching the Politics of Islamic Fundamentalism," *PS: Political Science and Politics*, vol. 31, no. 1 (March 1998): 52–59. The most sophisticated study that regards the system Khomeini created as having parallels to fascism is by Said Amir Arjomand, *The Turban for the Crown: The Islamic Revolution in Iran* (New York, 1988).

38. For an excellent analysis see Ramin Ahmadi, "Reading Postel on Tehran," Iranian.com (March 2, 2007), www.iranian.com/Ahmadi/2007/March/Postel/index.html

39. Masoud Kazemzadeh, "The State, Civil Society and the Prospects of Islamic Fundamentalism," *Comparative Studies of South Asia, Africa and the Middle East*, vol. 16, no. 1 (fall 1996).

40. Economic Research and Policy Department, Central Bank of the Islamic Republic of Iran, "Annual Review 1383 (2004/05), September 2005, www.cbi.ir/defaulten.aspx, cited in Elliot Hen-Tov, "Understanding Iran's New Authoritarianism," *The Washington Quarterly*, vol. 30, no. 1 (winter 2006–07): 172, 178.

41. Bill Samii, "Iran: Weak Economy Challenges Populist President," Eurasianet.org (July 23, 2006), www.eurasianet.org/departments/business/articles/pp072306.shtml

42. Daniel Pipes, "Unleash the Iranian Opposition [the Mujahedeen-e Khalq]," *New York Sun*, (July 10, 2007) reposted at http://www.danielpipes.org/pf.php?id = 4747; for an unusually candid and objective view of the PMOI see Daniel Pipes and Patrick Clawson, "[Mujahedeen-e Khalq:] A Terrorist U.S. Ally?" *New York Sun* (May 20, 2003) reposted at http://www.danielpipes.org/article/1100

43. http://iranpolicy.org/scholarsandfellows.php. Also see their site at www.iranpolicy.org

44. Iran Policy Committee, "U.S. Policy Options for Iran" (February 10, 2005), www.iranpolicy.org/uploadedFiles/USPolicyOptions_for_Iran_Feb2005.pdf

45. Masoud Kazemzadeh, "Ahmadinejad's Foreign Policy," *Comparative Studies of South Asia, Africa and the Middle East*, vol. 27, no. 2 (2007).

46. Kurt M. Campbell and Derek Chollet, "The New Tribalism: Cliques and the Making of U.S. Foreign Policy," *The Washington Quarterly*, vol. 30, no. 1 (winter 2006–07): 193–203. They identify four cliques in the Republican party: Oldsmobile Conservatives, Reagan Republicans, domestic-oriented America Firsters, and Faith Based Interventionists. They identify four groups in the Democratic party: Globalists, Truman Democrats, Come Home Americans, and American Skeptics.

47. Campbell and Chollet use the term "Reagan Republicans" for neoconservatives and "Truman Democrats" for liberal hawks. *The New Republic* is one of the publications that publish the views of liberal hawks. For Campbell and Chollet, the liberal hawk tradition goes back to President Truman, includes Senator Henry "Scoop" Jackson (D–Washington), and is currently represented by Senator Joseph Lieberman (I–Connecticut).

48. Peter Brookes, "Iran Is Interfering with Efforts to Build a Stable Iraq;" Reuel Marc Gerecht, "Diplomacy Is Not an Effective Option for Dealing with Iran;" Thomas Holsinger, "Military Force Is the Best Option for Dealing with Iran;" Terrence Henry, "Covert Action Could Be Used to Deal with the Iranian Nuclear Threat;" and Ilan Berman, "Encouraging an Internal Revolution Is a Viable Option for Dealing with Iran;" are all reprinted in Julia Bauder, ed., *Is Iran a Threat to Global Security?* (Detroit, 2006): 34–37, 58–64, 65–77, 78–83, and 84–96. For a typical neoconservative

position see Norman Podhoretz, "The Case for Bombing Iran: I hope and pray that President Bush will do it," *Opinion Journal* (*The Wall Street Journal* editorial page), May 30, 2007, www.opinionjournal.com/federation/feature/?id=110010139. For one of the most extreme neoconservative proposals see David Frum and Richard Perle, *An End to Evil: How to Win the War on Terror* (New York, 2003). For a thoughtful liberal hawk perspective see George Packer, ed., *The Fight Is for Democracy: Winning the War of Ideas in America and the World* (New York, 2003); Paul Berman, *Terror and Liberalism* (New York, 2004); and Paul Berman, "The Islamist, the Journalist, and the Defense of Liberalism," *The New Republic* (June 4, 2007).

49. Campbell and Chollet, "The New Tribalism." James Kurth uses the term "neoliberal" to refer to those whom Campbell and Chollet call "Globalist," for example, former Secretary of State Madeleine Albright and former UN ambassador Richard Holbrooke. See Kurth, "Ignoring History: U.S. Democratization in the Muslim World," *Orbis*, vol. 49, no. 2 (spring 2005).

50. James Kurth, "Global Threats and American Strategies: From Communism in 1955 to Islamism in 2005," *Orbis*, vol. 49, no. 4 (fall 2005).

51. Anatol Lieven and John Hulsman, *Ethical Realism: A Vision for America's Role in the World* (New York, 2006). Anatol Lieven, "The Iran We Have," *Open Democracy* (December 12, 2006), www.opendemocracy.net/democracy-irandemocracy/pahlavi_4152.jsp. Ray Takeyh, *Hidden Iran: Paradox and Power in the Islamic Republic* (New York, 2006). Gary Sick has been a long-time proponent of rapprochement with Iran; see Sick, "The United States and Iran: Truth and Consequences," *Contention: Debates in Society, Culture, and Science* (1996); interview with Sick at *Vaseteh: Journal of the European Society for Iranian Studies*, vol. 1, no. 1 (winter 2005); and Sick, "A Selective Partnership: Getting U.S.–Iranian Relations Right," *Foreign Affairs* vol. 85, no. 6 (Nov./Dec. 2006). This is a highly supportive review essay of Takeyh's book.

52. Barry Posen, "A Nuclear-Armed Iran: A Difficult But Not Impossible Policy Problem," The Century Foundation (December 6, 2006), www.tcf.org/list.asp?type=PB&pubid=596

53. Hoveyda, "Iran and America," *American Foreign Policy Interests*, vol. 28, no. 1 (February 2006): 15–21; Kurth, "Global Threats," op. cit.; Brookes, "Messing Up the Mullahs: Dubya's Covert Action Plan" (May 29, 2007), www.heritage.org/Press/Commentary/ed052907a.cfm; Brookes, "Iran: Our Military Options" (January 23, 2006), www.heritage.org/Press/Commentary/ed012306a.cfm; Brookes, "Iran Is Interfering with Efforts to Build a Stable Iraq," in Julia Bauder, ed., *Is Iran a Threat to Global Security?* (Detroit, 2006), originally published as "Facing the Facts About Iran" (August 23, 2005), www.heritage.org/Press/Commentary/ed082305b.cfm

54. Their Internet sites are www.ncafp.org, www.fpri.org; www.heritage.org, and www.washingtoninstitute.org. See especially the NCAFP's statements in this regard: "The Iranian Conundrum," *American Foreign Policy Interests*, vol. 28, no. 2 (April 2006): 159–161; and NCAFP, *Policy Statement on Iran and the United States: The Challenge of the Future* (March 15, 2002), www.ncafp.org/projects/middle_east/iran_us_mar02.pdf

55. See Marisa Morrison, "To Engage or Not to Engage?" National Interest online (December 29, 2006), www.nationalinterest.org/Article.aspx?id=13258

56. For an English translation of the constitution see www.oefre.unibe.ch/law/icl/ir00000_.html

57. Jim Saxton, "Reshaping our Iran Policy," National Interest online (January 3, 2007), www.nationalinterest.org/Article.aspx?id=13284

58. On this point see John Lewis Gaddis, *The Cold War: A New History* (New York, 2005).

59. Gary Sick, "A Bridge Too Far: A New Coordinated Policy Approach Against Iran,"

Iranian.com (January 22, 2007), www.iranian.com/Opinion/2007/January/GarySick110/index.html. Interview with Sick by Council on Foreign Relations' Bernard Gwertzman posted on January 23, 2007, at www.cfr.org/publication/12477. Jim Saxton, "Finally, An Iranian Containment Strategy," National Interest online (January 26, 2007), www.nationalinterest.org/Article.aspx?id=13508. Congressman Jim Saxton (R–New Jersey) is a member of the House Armed Services Subcommittee on Terrorism, Unconventional Threats, and Capabilities.

60. For example, Iranian Sunnis are forbidden to have a single mosque of their own in the capital, Tehran, a city of more than 10 million, and in Mashhad, the second largest city in Iran. The regime has also destroyed several Sunni mosques in Mashhad and in Zahedan (the largest city in the Sistan and Balochistan province). Many Sunni religious leaders have been assassinated by the regime's death squads, the most prominent being Mollah Rabii, the apolitical religious leader of the Sunni Kurds. Sunnis account for about 10 percent of Iran's population.

61. Sunni Kurds have historically exhibited Kurdish ethno-nationalism, whereas Shiite Kurds have strongly exhibited Iranian nationalism. Some top Iranian nationalist leaders have been Shiite Kurds such as Karim Sanjabi and Dr. Ali Ardalan, each of whom served as secretary general of the Iran National Front.

62. See John R. Bradley, "Iran's Ethnic Tinderbox," *The Washington Quarterly*, vol. 30, no. 1 (winter 2006–07): 181–190; Abbas William Samii, "Ethnic Tensions Could Crack Iran's Firm Resolve Against the World," *Christian Science Monitor* (May 30, 2006); and Massoud Ansari, "We Will Cut Them Until Iran Asks for Mercy," *London Telegraph* (January 15, 2006).

63. "Iran: Assassination, Confusion, or Disinformation?" *Stratfor Intelligence Briefing* (December 20, 2005) and Samii, "Ethnic Tensions."

64. Brenda Shaffer, "Iran's Volatile Ethnic Mix," *International Herald Tribune* (June 2, 2006) and Guy Dinmore, "U.S. Marines Probe Tensions Among Iran's Minorities," *Financial Times* (February 23, 2006).

65. This approach is also advocated by some antiappeasement realists such as Kurth. See Kurth, "Global Threats."

66. If the Swiss ambassador's notes are true, it may be more accurate to refer to the May 2003 roadmap as a "trial balloon" rather than a "grand bargain."

67. www.adelaideinstitute.org/2006December/contents_program1.htm

68. For some of Mr. Ramin's views see www.memri.org/bin/opener_latest.cgi?ID=SD140807

69. This direct quote is in Farsi from the BBC Persian service, available at www.bbc.co.uk/persian/iran/story/2006/12/061214_mf_holocaust.shtml. My translation.

70. The complete remarks were published in *Faslnameh Motaleat Rahbordi* (*Strategic Studies Quarterly*), which is the official publication of the Research Center of the Council for the Discernment of the Expediency of the System (Expediency Council for short). The members of the Expediency Council are appointed by the supreme leader and have several functions. One is to assist the supreme leader in providing general policies for the system. Another is to resolve disputes between the Majles (parliament) and the Council of Guardians when the Guardians declare that legislation passed by the Majles contradicts the constitution or sharia (Islamic divine law). Hojatolislam Hassan Rouhani is the former secretary of the Supreme National Security Council (SNSC) responsible for leading Iran's nuclear conflict with the outside world. He was also the head of the Research Center of the Expediency Council. After becoming president, Ahmadinejad succeeded in convincing the supreme leader to dismiss Rouhani. Ali Larijani succeeded him as secretary of the SNSC. Rouhani's remarks caused great controversy inside Iran where he was harshly attacked for revealing state secrets and

undermining Iran's case abroad. The site Baztab, for example, quoted "a high level expert of the nuclear file" as saying: "Why do we officially state that Iran deceived Europe and the IAEA and used dialogue as an excuse [to buy time] to advance its program?" An eight-page, single spaced excerpt of the original is available at www.iran-emrooz.net/index.php?/news/print/ 7046 (accessed February 22, 2006). The attack on Rouhani by Baztab is available at www. iran-emrooz.net/index.php?/nes2/print/7070/ (accessed February 23, 2006). Response from supporters of Rouhani from the Aftab newspaper's Internet site available at www.iran-emrooz.net/ index.php?/news2/print/7085/ (accessed February 24, 2006). Baztab is associated with General Mohsen Rezai who was the supreme commander of the Islamic Revolutionary Guards Corps (IRGC). Following the rise of Ahmadinejad and his fellow IRGC military commanders to power in 2005, a serious rift emerged between them and clerics associated with Rafsanjani. They blame one another for the various problems afflicting the regime. Rouhani is a cleric closely aligned with Rafsanjani. This conflict reached a new height in October 2006 with General Rezai who blamed Rafsanjani for convincing Ayatollah Khomeini to end the war with Iraq, thus preventing an Iranian victory. Rafsanjani responded by releasing Khomeini's private letter to the leaders of the regime wherein Khomeini used, as the reason for ending the war, the demand made by General Rezai concerning what he needed to win the war. Khomeini wrote: "The commander has said that we can have no victory for another five years, and even by then we need to have 350 infantry bridges, 2,500 tanks, 300 fighter planes, ... a considerable number of laser and **nuclear weapons** to confront the attacks." The official news agency ILNA, which had posted the letter on its Web site, removed the word *nuclear* within a few hours, reportedly after a call from the SNSC. It has been widely remarked that General Rezai and the IRGC have been the main advocates and sponsors of Iran's developing nuclear weapons, although various officials publicly deny that Iran had any desire for nuclear weapons or programs. See Nazila Fathi, "An Old Letter Casts Doubts on Iran's Goal for Uranium," *The New York Times* (October 5, 2006). There is concern by Rafsanjani and Rouhani that Ahmadinejad, Rezai, and other IRGC commanders are purposefully provoking the United States into a war.

71. Other issues that have raised suspicions of a secret weapons program include control of the program primarily in the hands of the IRGC, discovery of experimentations with Polonium 210, plans for hemispherical uranium castings, a missile program that makes most sense for delivering nuclear warheads, and the complete destruction of suspected facilities before allowing inspections. See Al J. Venter, *Iran's Nuclear Option: Tehran's Quest for the Atom Bomb* (Philadelphia, 2005).

72. For example, the fundamentalist regime explicitly asked Germany to swap a German tourist who had mistakenly strayed into Iranian waters for the man who assassinated four Iranian dissidents in Berlin in 1992. See "Diplomatic Wrangling: Iran Wants Germany to Swap Assassin for Jailed Tourist," in *Der Spiegel* (January 15, 2007), www.spiegel.de/international/0,1518,459731,00.html

73. Leverett's passage is somewhat vague. My interpretation is based on the assumption that Leverett is genuinely interested in human rights but chose his words poorly. The passage does allow an interpretation that Leverett simply wishes to use mere talk of human rights as a device to lure an important constituency to support his grand bargain. The entire passage is "To facilitate the implementation of internationally recognized human rights conventions and in parallel with Iran's human rights dialogue with the European Union, the Islamic Republic would commit to the commencement of an ongoing human rights dialogue with the United States, including representatives from nongovernmental organizations in both countries. (This commitment would help build

popular support for U.S.–Iranian rapprochement among important constituencies in both the United States and Iran.)," 23. The words in parentheses are by Leverett.

74. See Masoud Kazemzadeh and Shahla Azizi, "Life and Liberty: Political Culture and Regime Change in Iran," www.iranian.com (April 25, 2005), www.iranian.com/Opinion/2005/April/Regime/index.html

75. www.iranian.com/Poll/archives.php?poll_id=87

76. Although it may appear contradictory to Western eyes, Iranians are highly proud of their nationality, culture, and country although they strongly oppose their dictatorial government. See World Values Survey, 2000 table "Iran," in Patrick O'Neil, Karl Fields, and Don Share, eds., *Cases in Comparative Politics*, 2nd edition (New York, 2006), 339. President Bush's repeated praise of Iran's heritage, people, and culture while condemning the fundamentalist regime plays extremely well with the Iranian people and irritates the regime and its supporters.

77. BBC World Service poll is available at http://globalnin.com/branchedsurvey/results.aspx?surveyid=20&languageid=2&partnerid=0&isframed=False&branchid=0&filter=language

78. www.iranian.com/Poll/archives.php?poll_id=9

79. www.iranian.com/Poll/archives.php?poll_id=132

80. Thomas L. Friedman, "An American in Paris," *The New York Times* (January 20, 2005).

The sources of the Middle East's crises and American grand strategy

Masoud Kazemzadeh

ABSTRACT
This article argues that there are four major crises convulsing the Middle East. They are the Shia-Sunni conflict, rise of extremist militant fundamentalists, ethno-national demands, and pro-democracy movements. These have given rise to four clusters of actors. The article analyzes the ideological sources of Sunni and Shia fundamentalism, as well as Iran's grand strategy and American strategies and policies since 1979, trying to respond to these crises and challenges. It discusses the reasons for successes and failures of American policies and identifies lessons for future American policies toward the Middle East.

Introduction

According to the Chairman of the Joint Chiefs of Staff, Gen. Joseph Dunford, five major national security threats confront the United States: Iran, Sunni jihadi groups (e.g., al Qaeda and Islamic State of Iraq and Sham [ISIS]), North Korea, Russia, and China.[1] Each threat varies widely in nature, thus giving rise to a security environment far more complex than the one during the Cold War. Since the end of the Cold War, and particularly after 9/11, great debates on American grand strategy have resurfaced among scholars and practitioners. Some of these debates centered around the nature of the post–Cold Wat international system. Proponents argued whether the system was unipolar, multipolar, non-polar, or a clash of civilizations, among others.[2] After 9/11, these debates centered more around the most appropriate grand strategy, such as neoconservativism, restraint, selective engagement, and offshore balancing.[3]

The objective of this article is far more modest. I present an analysis of what are the main sources of the crises in the Middle East and what policies may worsen, contain, or abate the crises. The often-cited injunction by Sun Tzu—"Know the enemy and know yourself; in a hundred battles you will never be in peril"—has been a guiding principle for formulation of strategy for millennia.[4] In other words, a good strategy should contain an accurate diagnosis of the nature of the threat. This article presents an analysis of the nature of the conflict in the Middle East, the main actors, and policies that would affect the crises in positive or negative ways. It is hoped that such detailed and specific analyses of the crises in the Middle East may help explicate the nature of the threats and thus enrich discussions and debates on American grand strategy. The intention of this article is not to present a proposal for American grand strategy. Rather, the goal is to merely present, from the vantage point of the greater Middle East, the nature of the threats posed to the United States and the global system. The articulation of American grand strategy would rest upon analysis of other sources of threats (e.g., North Korea, Russia, China) and the nature of the international system, as well as American capabilities and political choices, which are beyond the purview of this article.

Grand strategy articulates a country's essential objectives (core interests, threats) and the means (plans, policies) to achieve those ends. According to Leonard Moffitt, grand strategy:

> correlates past, present, and potential crises, solutions, and trade-offs with the full panoply of problems, pressures, repercussions, and costs at various projections into the future. Its palette of resources, as well as its concerns, encompass much more than mere military force. It entails a systemic web of economic, cultural, historical, and geographical dynamics. Diplomacy, cultural and scientific interaction, and trade can exert as much influence on and in the changing global context of grand strategy as can armed might.[5]

For John Lewis Gaddis, grand strategy includes both tangible elements and intangible elements (e.g., psychology, culture, and perceptions of power relations). Gaddis argues:

> Grand strategy is as much about psychology as it is facts on the ground. The Bush administration intended that a demonstrated capacity for retaliation, pre-emption, and/or prevention in Afghanistan and Iraq would convince al Qaeda that the United States could not be run out of the Middle East. "Shock and awe" would dry up recruiting for the organization. And it would deter other states in the region and elsewhere from supporting terrorism in the future.[6]

Ideational factors such as ideology and culture, as well as perceptions of interests, have to be studied by scholars and strategists. As George Kennan's classic work clearly shows, a realistic and sophisticated grand strategy should be based upon a deep understanding of political and ideological conditions of the opponent. According to Kennan:

> The political personality of Soviet power as we know it today is the product of ideology and circumstances: ideology inherited by the present Soviet leaders from the movement in which they had their political origins, and circumstances of the power which they now have exercised for nearly three decades in Russia."[7]

Hence, one has to pay attention to the strategic culture. This may be more or less significant depending on the nature of the role of ideational factors for particular cases.

Four crises convulsing the Middle East

In order to understand the nature of the threat, one has to understand the ideology, culture, and interests of the various actors in the Middle East. Considering the saliency of Islamic fundamentalist movements, therefore one has to pay serious attention to the role of Islamic fundamentalist ideology on the strategic culture of these groups.[8] This article argues that the Middle East is going through at least four major phenomena, which are convulsing the region and beyond. First is the sectarian struggles between Sunnis and Shiites. The conflict began in the seventh century and has been going on intermittently ever since. The wars between the Sunni Ottomans and Shiite Iranians from the early sixteenth century to the late nineteenth century, as well as the Wahhabi attacks on Shiites from the eighteenth century, did not end with a conclusive victory for one side. Moreover, Shia and Sunni fundamentalists (e.g., Ayatollah Ruhollah Khomeini, Osama bin Laden, and Abubakr al-Baghdadi) have never accepted the principles of the Westphalian system such as the sanctity of international borders and noninterference in the internal religious affairs of another state. Khomeini, bin Laden and al-Baghdadi considered themselves the political leaders of people in many countries and thus they constructed political organizations to obey them and not the actual states they reside at. For example, the Lebanese Hezbollah considers the supreme leader of Iran to be its ultimate political leader. This means that the Lebanese Hezbollah would go to war or accept peace not by the order of the president of Lebanon but by the order of the supreme leader of Iran.[9]

Second, the rise of ultra-right-wing extremist militant fundamentalists (both Shia and Sunni) to power or prominence since 1979 has greatly increased violence and instability in the region. The emergence of contemporary Sunni fundamentalism goes back to the establishment of the Muslim Brotherhood in Egypt in 1928 by Hassan al-Banna.[10] There was further ideological articulation of the fundamentalist ideology by Seyyed Qotb, who was the Muslim Brotherhood's main theoretician, in the 1950s.[11] The Shia fundamentalists emerged in the late 1940s and early 1950s. The organization is called Fadaiyan Islam and the founder was Navab Safavi. The Shia fundamentalists borrowed heavily from, and modeled themselves on, the Muslim Brotherhood. The Shia fundamentalists adapted the Sunni fundamentalist ideology to Shia theological and clerical doctrines. Both Ayatollah Ruhollah Khomeini and Ayatollah Ali Khamenei have directly borrowed from the Muslim Brotherhood, Fadaiyan Islam,

Qotb, and Safavi.[12] Al Qaeda and ISIS, too, owe their ideological roots to the Muslim Brotherhood and Qotb. There is a misperception that al Qaeda and ISIS are directly related to the Wahhabi version of Islam. Actually, they are directly related to the Muslim Brotherhood and Qotb. The current leader of al Qaeda, Ayman al-Zawahiri, is not a Wahhabi, but he is a follower of Qotb. The same is true of the leader of ISIS, al-Baghdadi as well as of Abu Musab al-Zarqawi, the leader of al Qaeda in Iraq, which eventually became ISIS. To be a member of al Qaeda and ISIS, it is neither necessary nor sufficient to be a Wahhabi. However, to be in a leadership position in al Qaeda and ISIS, it is necessary to be a follower of Qotb. Hamas is the Palestinian affiliate of the Muslim Brotherhood. Its ideology comes from Banna and Qotb. Hamas's leaders and rank-and-file are not Wahhabis.

Third, the ethno-nationalist demands for a state of one's own by Kurds and Palestinians are major sources of intrastate and interstate tensions and crises. Modern nationalism is a product of Europe. Machiavelli, for example, wrote *The Prince* partly to promote the creation of one Italy out of many Italian-speaking principalities. After the French Revolution of 1789, nationalism became a major phenomenon, which gave rise to various ethno-nationalities demanding a nation-state of their own. The ethos of self-determination has proliferated the number of states in the state-centric Westphalian system. Not all of the new states have been regarded as legitimate by the people inhabiting them. Perhaps Iraq is the most extreme example of such a case. After the First World War, the British and the French created Iraq out of the territories of the Ottoman Empire.[13] The Kurds demanded a state of their own and briefly there was even a plan considering establishing such a state. However, the British, dismissing the wishes of local actors and wanting control of the oil fields, created the modern Iraq and placed a pliant ruler, Faisal, as king, who was compelled to grant a monopoly over the oil to the British.[14] The history of Iraq has been marred by numerous coups and terrible violence since.[15] The Kurdish struggle against the central government received great assistance from the United States, Israel, and the Shah of Iran between 1974 and 1975. Ever since 1974, the Kurdish Democratic Party of Iraq (KDPI) has established close relationships with the United States and Israel. Saddam Hussein pursued a policy that may be considered ethnic cleansing, if not genocide. According to Ariel Ahram, "about 100,000 Kurds [were] killed during the government's brutal dislocation campaign known as the Anfal."[16] Ahram adds:

> In the 1970s and 1980s, Saddam forcibly resettled or destroyed many Kurdish communities and encouraged Arab transmigration to the north to shift the demographic balance.... Persecution at Saddam's hands, including the genocidal razing of some four thousand villages in the late 1980s.[17]

After the 1991 war, when the U.S. defeated Saddam's forces in Kuwait, there were rebellions by the Shia in the south and the Kurds in the north. To prevent Saddam from killing even more Kurds, the U.S. established a no-fly zone over the Kurdish area. The Kurds then created the Kurdish Regional Government (KRG). During the 2003 U.S. invasion of Iraq, the Kurds closely cooperated with the U.S. The Kurdish political parties and the Kurdish people in Iraq have strongly supported the operations against Saddam. Since 2003, the U.S. government policy has been support for a unified federal Iraq and has opposed independence for KRG. The Kurds have gone along with the American wish, although the desire of their own population has been strongly for independence. The rise of ISIS, and the major role played by the Kurds, including capture of Kirkuk and its oil fields, which had historically been dominated by Kurds before Saddam's ethnic cleansing, have given rise to renewed demands by Kurds for a state of their own. The regime in Iran is strongly against independence for Kurds in Iraq and is reportedly engaged in activities to undermine and disrupt their efforts.[18] The government in Turkey has publicly opposed the idea, but due to close relations with the KRG and particularly with President Masoud Barzani of the KRG, it would probably go along with an independent Kurdistan in Iraq. Saudi Arabia has not made any public statement, but it would probably recognize the Kurdish state as a bulwark against Iran. Israel strongly supports independence for Kurdistan.

Fourth, the pro-democracy movements have been struggling against both the ruling authoritarian regimes and the fundamentalist forces. The Islamic fundamentalists (both Shia and Sunni) frame their jihad as the latest assertion of the 1,400-year-long war between the Christian world and Islam. The forces that oppose fundamentalists in the Islamic world have, instead, framed the Islamic fundamentalists as reactionary, misogynist, tyrannical threats to peace, security, and the welfare of the people in the region. Many pro-democracy and progressive academics, intellectuals, and political parties consider Islamic fundamentalists to be the Islamic world's equivalent to European fascism.[19] The fundamentalist and anti-fundamentalist forces in the Islamic world have been struggling for the hearts and minds of the people in the region. The pro-democracy movements, such as the Green Movement in Iran (2009–2010) and the Arab Spring, have shaken various states. Many Arab states were the creation of the British and French after WWI by the Sykes-Picot agreement and lack legitimacy in the eyes of many. Decades of pan-Arab and pan-Islamic agitation have further undermined the development of state legitimacy and "state-centered nationalism" (e.g., Iraqi nationalism, Libyan nationalism, Syrian nationalism, or Emirati nationalism). There is, however, unprecedented anti-Persian hatred and animosity among Arabs (at mass level as well as elite and state officials). Anti-Arab sentiments are also on the rise in Iran. Such sentiments are much higher today than they were during the Iran-Iraq war (1980–1988).

There are four major clusters of state and non-state actors in the Middle East and North Africa. One cluster of actors comprises the extremist Shia fundamentalists (the regime in Iran and Lebanon's Hezbollah) and their allies in Syria, Iraq, Yemen, Bahrain, and the Eastern Province of Saudi Arabia. A second cluster comprises pro-U.S. moderate authoritarian Arab Sunni states and their allies. The third set includes extremist Sunni fundamentalists such as ISIS and al Qaeda. The fourth set includes various pro-democracy groups and constituencies.

Iran's grand strategy

Ayatollah Khomeini's attempts in the early 1980s to overthrow the regimes in Iraq, Saudi Arabia, Kuwait, and Egypt was the primary cause of the Iran-Iraq war.[20] A broad coalition comprising secular nationalists (Iraq and Egypt) and conservative pro-U.S. monarchies (Saudi Arabia, Kuwait, the UAE, Qatar, Jordan, and Morocco) helped Saddam Hussein defeat Khomeini's attempt to export his revolution. Khomeini's "Last Will and Testament" is the foundational document of the regime's grand strategy where he tells Iran's officials and his supporters what they should do. Khomeini writes that only Shia Islam is true Islam and that Sunni are wrong. It goes on to viciously attack Wahhabi Islam and the Sunni leaders and calls upon the people to overthrow their regimes and to establish regimes like that of Iran's. Khomeini states:

> And more recently in order to eliminate the Quran and to secure the interests of the superpowers, the big satanic power. Through deviant governments of Islamic precepts, who falsely claim commitment to Islam, published the Quran with artful calligraphy and has distributed it throughout; it is to withdraw the Quran from the scene by this device ....
>
> We also see how, every year, king Fahd {[of Saudi Arabia} allocates large sums from the public wealth in order to publish [this kind of] Quran and to propagate anti-Quranic religion of Wahhabism—this utterly unfounded and superstitious cult—thereby attracting ignorant people and nations towards the superpowers and take [*sic*] advantage of noble Islam and the Holy Quran.
>
> ...And our nation, and also Islamic and oppressed nations of the world are proud that their enemy—who are the enemies of the glorious God, the Holy Quran and the noble Islam—are savages who would not hesitate to commit crimes and treacherous acts for their wicked and criminal goals and for obtaining domination and for satisfying their base interests [and in so doing], they recognize no enemy or friend.
>
> Chief among them, America this self-indulging terrorist, is a government which has enflamed the whole world and its ally is international Zionism, which, in order to satiate her desires will commit crimes which pens are embarrassed to enumerate and tongue likewise to describe; the silly notion of greater Israel lead them commit every conceivable crimes [*sic*]. Muslim nations and the oppressed people of the world are proud that their enemies are the Jordanian [king] Hussein, this professional vagrant criminal, and [king] Hassan {of Morocco} and Hosni Mubarak [of Egypt], the cohorts of Israel, are criminals and are in the service of America and Israel. [They] do not hesitate to commit any kind of treasons [*sic*] against their own nation.
>
> ...You oppressed masses of the world, you Muslim countries and you Muslims Rise to your feet and get your dues with your teeth and claws, defying the noisy propaganda of the superpowers, and expel the criminal men and the helm who give out the fruits of your toil to your enemies and the enemies of Islam, and let the self-committed and serving sectors of the society take the helm of your country, all joining together under the dignifying banner of Islam and rising against the enemies of Islam, marching towards an independent and free Islamic Republic and

resting assured that the realization of the proposition would mean the subjugation of all oppressors of the world, and helping the oppressed masses to become leaders and inheritors of your lands.[21]

What is understood in the Middle East, but not in the U.S. and Europe, is that Khomeini promoted a complex, extreme anti-Sunni policy. This policy was usually covert. Khomeini's Last Will and Testament is one of the few places where he openly explains his grand strategy. At the tactical level, however, Khomeini and his supporters have been willing to use Sunni groups whose policies at certain junctures benefit the objectives of the regime in Iran. There are many examples of the regime in Iran having transactional or instrumental relations with non-Shia groups. The regime in Iran has used HAMAS and Palestinian Islamic Jihad, two extremist Sunni groups, to attack Israel by providing them funds and weapons. As the bin Laden documents captured by the U.S. from the bin Laden compound and recently declassified by the Office of the Director of National Intelligence illustrate, the regime in Iran has provided a great deal of assistance to al Qaeda including safe passage of funds, operatives, and weapons.[22] As long as al Qaeda was attacking American and Saudi targets, Tehran was assisting them. Although officially Iran is an ally of the government of Afghanistan, Tehran has been covertly providing money, weapons, and training to the Sunni fundamentalist Taliban in Afghanistan as well as providing safe haven for their commanders inside Iran.[23] The goal has been to kill American troops and force the United States out of the region.[24] The regime in Iran has also used communist groups to further its own objectives. For example, Iran has provided assistance to communist Palestinian groups as well as to the PKK, the communist Kurdish group in Turkey. Providing tactical assistance to non-Shia groups has camouflaged the strategic anti-Sunni policy.

Today, Iran's grand strategy is designed by the Supreme Leader Ayatollah Ali Khamenei. Khamenei has argued that the post–Cold War international system will be characterized by the conflict between the West under American leadership and political Islam under the leadership of Iran.[25] Iran's regional strategy is formulated and carried out by the chiefs of the Islamic Revolutionary Guards Corps (IRGC) and the Qods Force (IRGC's elite foreign operations branch), after approval of the supreme leader. The chiefs of the IRGC and the Qods Force are Gen. Mohammad Ali Jafari and Gen. Ghassem Soleymani, respectively. Generals Jafari and Soleymani have stated that Iran's strategy is to create a bloc of Shia countries under the leadership of Iran.[26] These countries include Iraq, Syria, Lebanon, Bahrain, Yemen, and the Eastern Province of Saudi Arabia.

According to Gen. Soleymani:

The revival of Shia under the leadership of Iran creates a polarity and power for Iran, which has a political dimension and also a security dimension and also an economic dimension ....We know that three countries Iran, Saudi Arabia, and Iraq contain the most oil in the world. [Saudi] Arabia is first, Iran and Iraq are second and third, and that approximately 70 percent of the world's oil is located where the Shia live or about 80 percent is where the Shia live. Iraq's oil is in this corridor between Basra and Baghdad; Kuwait, and [Saudi] Arabia, which 80 percent of its oil is located in the Shia-populated places like Damam [and] Qatif, and it is also clear for Iran. The political leadership of Shiism exponentially adds to Iran's ethnic power. This assisted the Shia to recover their Shia sectarianism, which is one of the permanent legacies [of Ayatollah Khomeini]. If it were not for Iran, these events also would not occur.[27]

Soleymani adds that today Syria constitutes a major area of confrontation. On one side is Iran, and the other camp includes "the U.S., the Zionist regime, Turkey, and [Saudi] Arabia."[28] The "Saudis," Soleymani argues, "are afraid because [Khomeini's example and model] would have influence inside their country, and it will."[29] Since 1979, Iran's strategy has been to overthrow regimes in the region by the use of local proxies. Iran has been recruiting, training, funding, and arming various groups to overthrow the regimes in Iraq, Lebanon, Yemen, Bahrain, the Eastern Province of Saudi Arabia, and Kuwait.

American grand strategy and the Middle East

Since 1979, the United States has had two grand strategies available to deal with the region. The first grand strategy pursued alliance with the pro-U.S. Arab Sunni states and confrontation with Shia extremists. This was the American strategy between 1979 and 9/11. This strategy succeeded in containing Iran despite serious challenges from Saddam's invasion of Kuwait. After 9/11, the U.S. began confronting Sunni fundamentalists as well. The rise of Iran after the removals of the Taliban in Afghanistan and

Saddam in Iraq (as well as the 2008 economic downturn) greatly changed the balance of power in the region. By 2008, the costs in blood and treasure had made President Bush's strategy very unpopular among the American public and major segments of the foreign policy elites.

A second grand strategy is offshore balancing, whereby the balancer (e.g., the United States) would want to see a balance in which none of the actors achieves a decisive victory. The balancer would station its forces on ships and on bases away from the theater of operations. The balancer would not deploy boots on the ground unless the balance of power had changed and it would do so only temporarily. The strategy of offshore balancing is based on several assumptions. First, due to the conflict the antagonists on the ground would weaken and exhaust each other. Second, the balancer would assist the weaker side in order to prolong the conflict. Third, the decisive victory of any side would not be in the national interests of the balancer. Fourth, the balancer would be more powerful at the end of the conflict because it had not spent its blood and treasure in the conflict.[30] Offshore balancing was the grand strategy pursued by the British for much of the eighteenth and nineteenth centuries.

The Obama administration had pursued the offshore balancing strategy, as suggested in great detail by Christopher Layne.[31] In an interview with David Remnick, of *The New Yorker*, Obama said:

> And although it would not solve the entire problem, if we were able to get Iran to operate in a responsible fashion—not funding terrorist organizations, not trying to stir up sectarian discontent in other countries, and not developing a nuclear weapon—you could see an equilibrium developing between Sunni, or predominantly Sunni, Gulf states and Iran in which there's competition, perhaps suspicion, but not an active or proxy warfare.[32]

In another interview, Obama told Jeffrey Goldberg that Iran and Saudi Arabia should share the Middle East.[33] In actual practice, Obama had pursued the rapprochement with Iran and offshore balancing without Iran changing its aggressive policies. For example, Obama had pursued rapprochement with Iran, an actor that has had the upper hand and has menaced both the U.S. and the U.S. allies. According to the U.S. State Department, Iran is the number-one state sponsor of terrorism. Iran has succeeded in assisting Assad to defeat his opponents. Iran threatens the stability of pro-U.S. authoritarian Sunni regimes and provides lethal assistance to extremist groups attacking Israel. It also brutally suppresses the pro-democracy activists in Iran. The overthrow of the fundamentalist regime in Iran would be the greatest strategic victory for the U.S. since the collapse of the Soviet Union. The rapprochement with Iran while it has been pursuing such policies has further increased its power.

Moreover, President Obama also rejected the Clinton-Petraeus plan, which would have covertly provided major assistance to the Syrian moderate opposition forces.[34] At the time, the Assad regime was on the verge of collapse. Such a collapse would have caused a major strategic defeat for Iran. Hezbollah, Iran, and Russia have provided massive support to the Assad regime.

Due to Obama's offshore balancing policies (e.g., withdrawal of American troops from Iraq, lack of major support to anti-Assad forces since 2011, and rapprochement with Iran), ISIS came to control large areas of Iraq and Syria and gained the support of many Sunnis in the area and beyond. In other words, the antagonists hostile to the United States are stronger after than they were before Obama's policies went into effect. Since 1979, Iran has aggressively attempted to export its revolution. The Arab states of the Persian Gulf are fragile and vulnerable to Iranian subversion and aggression. Saddam's Iraq and the U.S. had deterred and contained Iran's threats. According to a 2015 report by Al Jazeera, Iran has in excess of 30,000 soldiers and advisers in Iraq. The report also stated that it is also believed that Iran has about 10,000 troops in Syria and has provided Assad billions of dollars in financial assistance.[35] It is estimated that Iran spends at least six billion dollars annually to keep Assad in power.[36] According to an American military source based in Iraq, Iran controls about 80,000 Shia paramilitary forces in Iraq, called Hashd al Shaabi, comprised primarily of Iraqi Shia, which Iran has organized, armed, trained and funded.[37] The Sunnis are petrified of Iran and its Shia allies in Iraq and Syria and have been providing assistance to extremists in order to counter Iran. Today, extremist Sunnis and extremist Shiites are stronger and moderate forces are weaker. The dynamics of the conflict have been such that the conflicts have not exhausted the extremists; rather the extremists have succeeded in mobilizing and galvanizing the Sunni and Shia populations to support them as the protectors of their respective communities. To put it another way, the fundamentalist regime in Iran, al Qaeda, and ISIS grew in strength after January 2009 due in large parts to Obama's policies.

The Obama administration did not do anything to help Ayad Allawi (a moderate, pro-U.S. secular Shia with close alliances with the Sunnis), who received the highest number of votes and could have formed a government while Iran went full throttle to pressure Kurdish parties and other groups to form a coalition with Nouri Maliki, Iran's ally. It was Maliki's extreme repression of Sunnis (many of whom had been working with the U.S.) that drove many of them into support of (or acquiescence toward) ISIS. The dynamics were predictable. Obama withdrew American troops from Iraq, Iran filled the vacuum, Maliki and Iran pursued a terribly discriminatory policy toward the Sunnis. ISIS gained great support from Sunnis in order to defend themselves from Shia extremists. Although the Sunnis are a minority in Iraq (about 20 percent), they are the overwhelming majority of Muslims around the world (about 85 to 88 percent).

In neighboring Syria, the majority Sunni Arabs (about 60 to 65 percent) have been oppressed by the Alawite Assad's regime. Alawites constitute about 12 percent and the Shia are about 3 percent of the population in Syria. In Syria, while Iran provided Bashar Assad with billions of dollars, IRGC's Qods force fighters, and thousands of Lebanese Hezbollah fighters, Obama refused to support the Clinton-Petraeus plan. Even after numerous uses of chemical weapons against civilians by Assad, there was no military action against his forces by Obama. Even after Assad's repeated use of chloride bombs and barrel bombs, the Obama administration did not use military strikes against Assad's forces. Only in 2015 did the Obama administration provide small amounts of light arms and training to the opposition, which was too little too late. And under Obama's policy, the Pentagon demanded that the Syrian fighters sign a pledge that they would fight only against ISIS (and not Assad's forces). Therefore, the rise of ISIS is the direct result of Obama's polices toward Iran, Iraq, and Syria.

Bahrain and Saudi Arabia are especially vulnerable due to the affinity of their Shia populations with the Shia fundamentalist regime in Iran. A Sunni king rules Bahrain though Sunnis constitute about 30 percent of the population and Shia comprise about 70 percent. About 10 to 15 percent of the population is of Persian descent. More than 85 percent of the Saudi population is Sunni. About 10 to 15 percent of Saudi Arabia is Shia, and the overwhelming majority of them live in the Eastern Province. According to one source, the Shia living in the Eastern Province are about two million, constituting about 12 percent of the country's population.[38] Much of Saudi oil is located in this province. There are close tribal and kin relations between the Shia in Bahrain and the Eastern Province. Since the early 1980s, Iranian government has been recruiting, training, funding, and arming Shia from Bahrain and the Eastern Province. Iran has already helped establish the so-called Saudi Hezbollah, which according to the FBI was responsible for the Khobar Towers attacks on June 25, 1996, that killed nineteen American military personnel.[39]

Obama's rapprochement with Iran unraveled the balance of power in the region. Obama's policy of rapprochement with Iran's Supreme Leader Ayatollah Ali Khamenei has not made Khamenei stop expanding Iran's influence in Iraq, Syria, Lebanon, Yemen, and Bahrain. There is no reason to believe that with the further disengagement of American power from the region, Khamenei would not attempt to expand Iran's influence into Bahrain and Saudi Arabia's Eastern Province.

Obama's policies toward other countries in the region further aggravated the situation. In Lebanon, the Obama administration's hands-off policy caused several parties (the Druze and some Christians) to leave Saad Hariri's moderate pro-U.S. government and side with the coalition supported by Hezbollah, Iran's proxy. Complaints by top American military officials about the killings of American military personnel in Iraq and Afghanistan by Iran and its proxies were met with lack of retaliation by Obama. There was no serious retaliation when a plot was discovered that the IRGC was involved in a plan to assassinate the Saudi ambassador to the United States in Washington. When one of America's most sophisticated spy drones landed in Iran, Obama overrode the decision of the commanders to either bomb the drone or send a team to salvage it.

Obama had sent at least five secret letters to Khamenei expressing his respect and recognition of the fundamentalist regime and promising that he would not pursue regime change. Obama also ended U.S. financial assistance to Iranian human rights groups that would merely document human rights violations by the regime. In the words of Eli Lake, "Obama from the beginning of his presidency tried to turn the country's ruling clerics from foe to friends. It was an obsession."[40]

When Khamenei used massive violence to suppress the pro-democracy movement in Iran in 2009, the pro-democracy protesters publicly asked: "Obama, are you with the regime or with us?" There was a demoralizing silence from Obama. According to Jay Solomon's book, *The Iran Wars*, the CIA was ordered by Obama not to do anything that would undermine Khamenei's hold on power during the mass uprisings in 2009–2010. In Solomon's words, "The Agency has contingency plans for supporting democratic uprisings anywhere in the world. This includes providing dissidents with communications, money, and in extreme cases even arms."[41] Solomon adds, "But in this case the White House ordered it to stand down."[42]

Obama's policy of rapprochement with Khamenei meant distancing the U.S. from its allies such as Saudi Arabia, Israel, Kuwait, Jordan, and Egypt, as well as giving in to many of Khamenei's demands and overlooking Iran's expansionist policies in the region. These concessions include undermining the consensus on zero uranium enrichment by the fundamentalist regime on Iranian soil, a consensus that included six major UN Security Council (UNSC) resolutions supported by Russia and China as well as the EU. These UNSC resolutions were Chapter 7 resolutions, which considered the regime a threat to peace and security of the world. Obama even gave up real, thorough investigations of the past weaponization program as well as current concerns such as inspections on Parchin by IAEA inspectors to all the suspect locations. These major concessions to Khamenei were put into a secret side agreement between the IAEA and the Iranian government and not into the official public accord, a tactic that successfully hid the concessions from the U.S. Congress until it was discovered much later.[43] The accord allows the regime to keep the nuclear infrastructure, including over 6,050 centrifuges, Fordow site deep into a mountain, and all the research and development of centrifuges (e.g., IR-8) that enrich about eight to twenty times the current ones. Obama also released agents and collaborators of the fundamentalist regime responsible for illegal exports of nuclear and missile technology to Iran who were in American prisons, under trial, or sought by the Interpol. The magnitude of this concession came to light in an investigative report by Politico in April 2017.[44]

The nuclear deal was terribly in favor of the fundamentalist regime; so much so that even the French objected to the concessions during the negotiations. According to a leaked document published by the Associated Press, a secret side agreement was placed within the secret IAEA-Iran agreement instead of the body of the publicly disclosed agreement between Iran and the P5 + 1. Both the Iranian government and the U.S. have confirmed the authenticity of the leaked document.[45] According to the secret side agreement, from year 11, Iran can replace 5,060 old centrifuges with between 2,500 and 3,500 modern centrifuges that are five times more efficient. This secret agreement allows Iran to reduce the breakout time from about 12 months to less than six months.[46]

Despite the extensive concessions that the Obama administration gave Iran, the fundamentalist regime has violated its commitments. The Obama administration official in charge of monitoring Iran's implementation of the nuclear agreement, Ambassador Stephen Mull, testified in Congress that Iran has fully complied with the agreement. Unfortunately, his testimony does not appear to be the truth.[47] The agreement explicitly requires that Iran acquire all nuclear related materials through a channel established for such purpose. Two official reports released by German intelligence agencies in June 2016 present explicit evidence that Iran repeatedly has violated its commitments. The German federal internal security agency (BfV) released its annual report, which states that Iran's "illegal proliferation-sensitive procurement activities in Germany registered by the Federal Office for the Protection of the Constitution persisted in 2015 at what is, even by international standards, a quantitatively high level. This holds true in particular with regard to items which can be used in the field of nuclear technology."[48]

The German intelligence body in the state of North Rhine-Westphalia added that during 2015, Iran had made 141 attempts to purchase nuclear and missile technologies, "ninety" of which were attempts to "procure technology that could be used for the development of nuclear weapons and launchers."[49] German intelligence states that they succeeded in thwarting about 90 percent of Iran's attempts.[50] In 2014, Iran had made 83 similar attempts, which the BfV states indicates a major increase in Iran's illegal activities after the nuclear agreement was reached. The German intelligence further states that these illegal procurements were usually made "by Iranian strawmen and shell companies through China, Turkey, and the United Arab Emirates."

The Institute for Science and International Security has released a report about Iran stating that it has made attempts to procure tons of carbon fiber, an item used for building centrifuge rotors. Iran already has sufficient amounts for several years for its centrifuges under the parameters of the nuclear agreement.[51] This violation may indicate that Iran may have a clandestine program for the manufacture of centrifuges so that it can enrich uranium outside the purview of the IAEA.

The IAEA test results of samples taken from the Parchin military site in fall 2015 showed the presence of "chemically man-made particles of natural uranium."[52] For American officials, this was evidence of experimentation related to a nuclear bomb. However, neither the IAEA nor the P5 + 1 is pressing for taking more samples or visits by the IAEA inspectors. This is highly significant because Iran had refused for more than two years repeated requests by the IAEA to visit the site while it was making major modifications to the site. Further sampling is necessary to conclusively establish the presence of uranium. The IAEA and the U.S. are not pressing for re-sampling or visits because they fear that Iran would refuse.

The State Department spokesman took great pains to attempt to respond to journalists who asked about some of these revelations.[53] The beleaguered spokesman kept repeating the talking points that the U.S. does not have any indication that Iran has violated its obligations under the nuclear agreement. What is clear is that the Iranian regime has continued its clandestine nuclear weapons program despite the agreement reached on July 14, 2015.

There might have been good reasons for the Obama administration officials to overlook the facts. First, a public acknowledgement of Iran's cheating would have unraveled the agreement. Second, the unraveling of the agreement would have resulted in Iran expelling the IAEA inspectors and expedited the nuclear weapons program. There was not enough time to utilize economic sanctions to stop the breakout. Clearly, the Obama administration lacked credibility in making threats of military strikes after the administration's refusal to enforce its red lines when Assad used chemical bombs against civilians. With the evaporation of Obama's military deterrence, the actual use of military strikes was the only option left to stop Iran's nuclear bomb, an option President Obama did not wish to use. Thus, by ignoring Iran's violations, it was hoped that Iran would proceed slowly, which would allow the Obama administration to postpone a forceful response to the next president. The Trump administration's threat of force might be the only option other than actual military strikes to convince Ayatollah Khamenei to stop going nuclear.[54]

Obama's offshore balancing makes two further assumptions: (1) without American leadership and major role, regional actors would have to step up and counter Iran; and (2) when they do, their actions would be in America's national interests. In actuality, however, many small states are too weak to step up. Without American support, it is not rational for Kuwait, the UAE, Qatar, or Jordan to stand up to Iran. And when other states have stepped up, their actions have not been consistent with American interests. For example, Israel began a program of assassinations of Iran's nuclear scientists. The Obama administration strongly opposed the Israeli actions and stopped them. The Obama administration had also opposed Israeli military strikes on Iran's nuclear facilities. Many other states also looked the other way when many extremist Sunni jihadi groups recruited and/or transited through their territories to reach Syria and Iraq. The Turkish government has been more concerned about the rise of Kurdish power (in Syria and Turkey) than that of ISIS. Much of Turkey's firepower has targeted the Kurdish groups, many of whom have been cooperating with the U.S.

Obama's offshore balancing strategy had clearly failed. Unlike in 2009, by January 2017 the Shia fundamentalist regime in Iran was far more secure. And the opposition forces were badly demoralized. The regime also has far more influence in Arab countries than ever before. Not fearful of Obama's retaliation, the regime was also much more aggressive in Syria, Iraq, Yemen, and Bahrain, and pursued its policies much more overtly. Obama's policy of rapprochement with Khamenei had managed to alienate Arab allies (Saudi Arabia, Kuwait, the UAE, Jordan, Egypt, and Algeria), antagonize Israel, confuse Turkey, demoralize the Iranians who oppose the fundamentalist regime, and stabilize the fundamentalist regime in Iran. The ISIS, which is far more extreme than al Qaeda, had actually succeeded in establishing a functioning state in a large landmass in Iraq and Syria and its affiliates control landmasses in Libya, northern Nigeria, and the Sinai Peninsula, as well as influence in Yemen and Afghanistan.

The Trump administration and the Middle East

In contrast to the Obama administration, President Trump and his national security team are pursuing a policy of standing up to the fundamentalist regime. On May 21, 2017, Trump gave a major speech in Riyadh to a large gathering of states organized by Saudi Arabia. Trump proposed a broad coalition to counter and fight radical Islamic terrorism. He named these terrorist entities to include the fundamentalist regime in Iran, Lebanese Hezbollah, ISIS, al Qaeda, and Hamas.[55] According to Secretary of Defense Gen. Mattis, "Everywhere you look, if there's trouble in the region, you find Iran ....The nations in the region and others elsewhere are trying to checkmate Iran and the amount of disruption, the amount of instability they can cause."[56] Secretary of State Rex Tillerson has stated:

> The JCPOA fails to achieve the objective of a non-nuclear Iran; it only delays their goal of becoming a nuclear state. This deal represents the same failed approach of the past that brought us to the current imminent threat we face from North Korea. The Trump administration has no intention of passing the buck to a future administration on Iran ....The evidence is clear. Iran's provocative actions threaten the United States, the region, and the world.[57]

Other principles such as Vice President Mike Pence, National Security Adviser Gen. H. R. McMaster, CIA Director Mike Pompeo, and Secretary of Homeland Security Gen. John Kelly also hold strong views on Iran.[58]

In mid-April, President Trump ordered a 90-day review of Iran policy.[59] By mid-June, elements of the policy included: (1) repairing alliances with America's allies in the region; (2) countering Iran's expansionist and destabilizing efforts in Iraq, Syria, Yemen, Bahrain, and Saudi Arabia; (3) reimposing sanctions for missile tests and human rights violations; and (4) at a minimum, strict enforcement of the nuclear accord with Iran and a possible termination of the accord after the ninety-day review. The interagency review was not ready by 90 days. The first version of the strategy was presented by President Trump on October 13, 2017. It contained all the elements mentioned above. Trump did not declare the IRGC a foreign terrorist organization but did order the Treasury Department to impose sanctions on it for terrorist activities. Trump declined to certify that Iran was compliant with the nuclear deal; however, he did not declare the U.S. would be leaving the JCPOA. Trump gave Congress 90 days to try to either fix the deal or leave the deal and re-impose sanctions that had been suspended under the deal. By January 15, 2018, Congress had not taken any actions on the JCPOA. In January, Trump released a major policy statement that gave Congress (and European allies) another 90 days to come up with ways to revise the deal or he would leave the deal. In other words, Trump did not leave the deal. Most significantly, he continued the suspension of the sanctions that the JCPOA was based on. Trump said that this was the last time that he would do so. The Treasury added more individuals and companies to the sanctions list.

The Iranian people are far more democratic, liberal, progressive, modern, secular, pluralistic, tolerant, and pro-American than the fundamentalist regime ruling them. The primary obstacle to democracy, freedom, and human rights in Iran is the fundamentalist regime. Regime change in Iran will not only have wonderful benefits for the Iranian people but also will bring positive results for the region and the world.

Both the Saudi government and the Shia fundamentalist regime are terribly authoritarian and reactionary. However, their domestic dynamics and their foreign policies are very different. Saudi Arabia is an ultra-conservative, status quo power. The Shia fundamentalist regime is a revisionist power attempting to export its ultra-reactionary form of government to the region and undermine the international system using extremist violent proxies.

In order to promote American national interests, the interests of the Iranian and Saudi people, as well as the values of democracy, human rights, and freedom, the wisest policy would be to first pursue regime change in Iran, and after the accomplishment of that goal, then promote gradual liberalization, reform, and democratization in Saudi Arabia.

Unless the current trends are halted, the extremist Sunni and Shia fundamentalist forces will continue their advances and undermine the stability and security of the region and beyond. Drastic changes in American policies toward the Middle East may be the best way, if not the only way, to reverse the current trends. A new grand strategy may have to include the following policies. First, the U.S. policy toward Iran should be regime change, not rapprochement.

Second, the U.S. should support the Kurdish demand in Iraq for an independent state of their own. The Kurdistan Regional Government has set September 25, 2017, for a referendum on independence. That policy would, in all likelihood, result in disintegration of Iraq into three independent states for Kurds, Shia Arabs, and Sunni Arabs. This is probably the best way to stop the Shia oppression of the Sunni population, and thus undermine ISIS or other future extremist Sunni groups. Although ISIS would be defeated sooner or later, as long as the Shia majority in Iraq oppress the Sunni minority, the Sunnis would find ways to resist. Considering that Sunnis comprise over 85% of all the Muslims in the world, there are plenty of Sunnis willing to go to Iraq to assist their fellow Sunnis. The Sunnis and Shiites will be fighting for some time to come. The U.S. should support the moderate forces in both camps.

The Kurdish state will be democratic, stable, pluralistic, and pro-American. The existence of a democratic, multiparty, prosperous country in the region would have great positive effect on the pro-democracy forces in the greater Middle East. Moreover, the Kurdish state will be a reliable strategic partner for the United States. Fearful of the fundamentalist regime in Iran and the Turkish government, the Kurds in Iraq would likely be very happy to provide the U.S. military bases on their soil. The Kurdish population of KRG is about five million. Turkey's population is about 80 million, about 19 percent of whom are Kurds.[60] Between 1984 and 1999, the conflict caused about 35,000 deaths among PKK fighters, local population, and security forces, as well as costing the economy about $120 billion.[61] Violent conflict between the PKK and the Turkish government has flared up again after a long hiatus. The KRG President Masoud Barezani has very good relations with Ankara and opposes the PKK. American troops already use bases in the KRG. American military presence would serve as deterrence against threats from Iran and Turkey.

The creation of an independent Kurdistan in Iraq will greatly undermine the Shia regime in Iran. Iran's population is about eighty-two million.[62] Kurds constitute about 8 to 10 percent of Iran's population. About 40 percent of Iranian Kurds are Shia and they live in the province of Kermanshah. The Shia Kurds have been strongly against the fundamentalist regime and for Iranian nationalism and secular democracy. Since 1949, the Shia Kurds have strongly supported Iran National Front (INF), which was established by Dr. Mossadegh. The INF has been Iran's main pro-democracy political party (to be more precise a coalition of parties and individuals). The number-one leader of the INF in the late 1970s and early 1980s was Dr. Karim Sanjabi, who was a Shia Kurd. After Sanjabi, the number-one leader of the INF was Dr. Ali Ardalan, who was also a Shia Kurd. In 1980, for the first election for the *Majles* after the revolution, both Sanjabi and Ardalan won in their constituencies. The fundamentalists threatened to kill them if they came to Tehran to take their parliamentary seats. Sanjabi escaped Iran in 1981 and came to the U.S. Ardalan was severely tortured to force him to falsely confess to spying for the U.S. He refused to do so and suffered two heart attacks under torture. Many leaders and members of the INF were executed or assassinated by the fundamentalists, including Khosrow Qashqai, who was executed for being a member of the INF and having won a seat for the *Majles* in 1980.

The Sunni Kurds comprise about 60 percent of Iranian Kurds and live mostly in northern parts of the Kermanshah province, Kurdistan province, and the western parts of the Western Azerbaijan province. Kurdish ethno-nationalists draw their support from among the Sunni Kurds. The largest such party is the Democratic Party of Iranian Kurdistan (DPIK). Although the party began as a far-left party close to the Soviet Union during the 1940s, under the able leadership of Dr. Abdol Rahman Ghassemlou it gradually became a pro-Western party after 1979. It has been working closely with both the U.S. government and the KRG. The agents of the Iranian government (IRGC and the Ministry of Intelligence) assassinated Dr. Ghassemlou and two of his lieutenants in Vienna on July 13, 1989.[63] The Iranian government also assassinated Dr. Sadegh Sharafkandi (Ghassemlou's successor), along with two of his lieutenants with another Iranian progressive, in Berlin on September 17, 1992.[64] According to data provided by the DPIK, the Iranian government was responsible for the killing of over 40,000 Kurdish civilians in indiscriminate bombings of residential areas as well as completely destroying or totally depopulating hundreds of Kurdish villages.[65] Under the able leadership of Mostafa Hejri, the DPIK has brought other Iranian Kurdish parties closer together in the past several years. It has also expanded its activities inside Iranian Kurdistan. The DPIK has announced that it would not attack any targets inside Iran but it would defend itself. And when the IRGC made several attacks on them, the DPIK Peshmargas engaged them in self-defense and killed several IRGC attackers.

Despite massive repression by the fundamentalist regime, Iranian Kurds continue to resist. The regime is worried that independence for Kurds in Iraq will further galvanize and encourage Iranian Kurds.

Third, the U.S. should pursue the Clinton-Petraeus plan and massively support the moderate opposition to overthrow the Assad regime. Some worry that American assistance to the moderate opposition or partition of Iraq might lead to partition of Syria. The status quo is not in the interests of the U.S. or that of the majority of the Syrian people. Assad is in power due to the massive intervention of Iran, Lebanese Hezbollah, and Russia. Even with such support and massive violence, still Assad and his allies do not control much of the territory and the people. A rump Alawite state would protect the Alawite population from retribution from the victims of Assad's policies, as well as provide naval and air bases to Russia. A Sunni Arab state would be a viable state and it might want to merge with the Sunni Arab state in present-day Iraq. Like Iraq, Syria was the creation of the French and British after the First World War. After so much intercommunal violence, it appears most unlikely that the various ethno-sectarian communities could peacefully coexist. Partition of Syria might be the only solution for ending the civil war.

Fourth, the U.S. should repair the alliance with the Arab Sunni allies. They had lost trust and confidence in American support in the struggle against Iran and extremist Shia forces. The Trump administration has already greatly repaired the relationship with Saudi Arabia, the UAE, and Egypt. The U.S. should reach a quid pro quo with these allies: in exchange for American policy of regime change in Iran, they would prevent all assistance to extremist Sunni forces in Syria, would send massive assistance to Syrian moderates, and once moderates emerge in Iraq they would send assistance to them and would promise to change their discriminatory policies toward the Shiites in their own countries. The American, Muslim, Arab summit in Riyadh in May 2017 went a long way toward this goal.

Conclusion

As the wealthiest and most powerful country in the world, the U.S. is the only country that can orchestrate a broad global coalition to isolate and defeat both Shia and Sunni extremists. Without a farsighted policy by the U.S., the region is headed toward a sectarian bloodbath, interstate wars, and collapse of oil-rich states. The ongoing Sunni-Shia sectarian wars in Syria and Iraq could easily spread to Saudi Arabia, Bahrain, Lebanon, Kuwait, Qatar, and the UAE. The rivalry and proxy wars between Iran and Saudi Arabia have escalated in the aftermath of Obama's nuclear deal with Iran. From late 2015 to early 2017, Iran's top military officials were making explicit threats of military strikes against Saudi Arabia, threats that had not been heard since the early 1980s. In 2009, Obama was praising Erdogan's Turkey as a role model. Today Turkey is lurching toward authoritarianism and instability.

Unless there is a reversal of Obama's offshore strategy, we should expect regional wars involving not only states such as Iran, Turkey, Israel, Saudi Arabia, Kuwait, Jordan, and Bahrain, but also drastic growth of transnational Sunni movements (e.g., ISIS, al Qaeda) as well as Shia extremist groups (Hezbollah, Shia extremist violent forces in Iraq). Trump's policies have in fact made major reversals of Obama's policies. They have been steps in the right direction.

The crises and upheavals in the Middle East predated Obama's presidency, but Obama's policies greatly worsened the crises. Had Obama kept 10,000 troops in Iraq and opposed al-Maliki's anti-Sunni chauvinist policies, there would be no ISIS as such. Had Obama assisted the Syrian moderate opposition in 2011 and pursued active regime change, there likely would not be over 400,000 dead Syrians and over 9.5 million refugees. Syria's tragedy may become a prelude to much more of the same in the region. And all of these will pale in comparison if and when the fundamentalist regime ruling Iran completes its nuclear weapons program.

The direct Russian military intervention in September 2015 in Syria and its alliance with one cluster of actors (the Shia extremist regime in Iran, Hezbollah, and their allies in Iraq and the Assad regime) and opposition to three other clusters have clearly exposed the failures of Obama's offshore balancing strategy. Historically, major events have compelled presidents to reconsider their grand strategies.[66] For example, the Soviet invasion of Afghanistan made President Carter place his earlier pursuit of human rights in pro-American dictatorial regimes on the back burner and declare the Carter Doctrine, which stated that the Persian Gulf was an American vital interest and that the U.S. would go to war to protect its interest, a clear signal to the Soviets that the U.S. would not tolerate Soviet invasion of Iran or Pakistan. The 9/11 terrorist attacks made President George W. Bush change his earlier conventional realist grand strategy, which regarded the rise of China as the main threat to American interests, to a neoconservative one that regarded the international system to be unipolar with American primacy, one in which the U.S. enjoyed such preponderance of power that it could easily impose its will, and with little costs to overthrow various rogue regimes and establish stable democratic regimes in countries with little or no histories of democratic rule.[67]

President Obama considers his Middle East strategy a success.[68] Although Hillary Clinton had closely embraced many of Obama's domestic policies, she has distanced herself from many of Obama's Middle East policies. For example, Clinton: (1) supports a no-fly zone and safe zones in Syria; (2) supports increased assistance to Syria's moderate opposition; (3) emphasizes strict enforcement of the nuclear deal with Iran (whereas many believe that the Obama administration overlooked Iran's violations of the nuclear accord); (4) considers lack of support for the 2009 protests in Iran a mistake; (5) supports pro-democracy and human rights activists in Iran; (6) advocates close relations with Israel (a subtle reminder of the strained relations between the Obama administration and the Israeli government); and (7) advocates repairing the strained relations with America's moderate Sunni Arab allies (e.g., Saudi Arabia, Egypt, and Jordan).[69] Moreover, Clinton strongly supports reauthorization of sanctions because the current ones expire by the end of 2016, which would allow the U.S. government to snap back to these sanctions when the U.S. decides to reimpose them due to Iran's violations of the nuclear accord.[70] The officials of the Obama administration did not voice support for such reauthorization. After its passage by Congress by overwhelming margins, Obama did not veto the bill and allowed the bill to become law without his signature. Clinton's spokesman stated to *The Hill*, "As president, she will also continue to enforce, and strengthen as necessary, sanctions on Iran's support for terrorism, human rights abuses and ballistic missile activity."[71]

There is a general consensus among observers that Clinton's Middle East policy is tougher than that of Obama's.[72] Many leading Democratic members of Congress have also strongly opposed Obama policies toward Iran. For example, four prominent Democratic senators (Chuck Schumer, Robert Menendez, Ben Cardin, and Joe Manchin) and 25 House Democrats voted against the nuclear deal. There has also been vociferous opposition by leading Republicans in Congress to Obama's policies toward Iran and Syria. These indicate that in 2017 those at the highest levels of decision making have realized the necessity of new grand strategies for the Middle East. Trump's national security team, thus, has had great support in Congress for formulating strong policies toward the Middle East.

This article has identified four major phenomena convulsing the Middle East as well as the four major clusters of actors that are pursuing their objectives and responding to those phenomena. The U.S. and other powers have to investigate what constitutes their core national interests in the Middle East and formulate their grand strategies accordingly. Obama's strategy had clearly failed. A new American grand strategy is necessary to create a new security structure in the Middle East. Some scholars of the international system believe that we are entering a multipolar international system, and thus the U.S. simply lacks the power (economic, military, or diplomatic) to have real influence around the world and therefore it would be better to avoid conflicts in which the U.S. is destined to lose.[73] Other scholars argue that, whether we still have a unipolar international system or are gradually entering a multipolar system, the U.S. is not only the most powerful military and economic force in the world, but will remain so for many years to come.[74] If the latter group is right, then a more sophisticated grand strategy by the U.S. may be the best hope the U.S. and the region have in resolving the crises in the Middle East. If the former group is right, then the world is entering a prolonged and bloody period of conflicts emanating from the Middle East.

Notes

1. Jim Garamone, "Dunford Details Implications of Today's Threats on Tomorrow's Strategy," DOD News, August 23, 2016, https://www.defense.gov/News/Article/Article/923685/dunford-details-implications-of-todays-threats-on-tomorrows-strategy/ (accessed June 15, 2017). I use "ISIS" to refer to the group that has been variously referred to by ISIS, ISIL (Islamic State of Iraq and Levant), and IS (Islamic State). The term "Sham" that the group uses is an old term that refers to greater Syria, which includes Syria, Lebanon, and parts of Jordan, Israel, and Palestine. Some use the word "Daesh," which is the Arabic acronym of ISIS. The core of ISIS in Iraq was called al Qaeda in Iraq or Al Qaeda in Mesopotamia.
2. Charles Krauthammer, "The Unipolar Moment," *Foreign Affairs* 70, no. 1 (1990): 23–33; William C. Wohlforth, "The Stability of a Unipolar World," *International Security* 24, no. 1 (Summer 1999): 5–41; Charles W. Kegley, Jr., and Gregory A. Raymond, "Must We Fear a Post–Cold War Multipolar System?" *Journal of Conflict Resolution* 36, no. 3 (September 1992): 573–585; Richard N. Haass, "The Age of Nonpolarity: What Will Follow U.S. Dominance," *Foreign Affairs* 87, no. 3 (May/June 2008): 44–56; and Samuel P. Huntington, "The Clash of Civilizations," *Foreign Affairs* 72, no. 3 (Summer 1993): 22–49.
3. David Frum and Richard Perle, *An End to Evil: How to Win the War on Terror* (New York: Ballantine Books, 2004); Barry Posen, *Restraint: A New Foundation for U.S. Grand Strategy* (Ithaca, NY: Cornell University Press, 2014); Robert J. Art, "Geopolitics Updated: The Strategy of Selective Engagement," *International Security* 23, no. 3 (Winter 1998–99): 79–113; and Christopher Layne, "From Preponderance to Offshore Balancing: America's Future Grand Strategy," *International Security* 22, no. 1 (1997): 86–124.
4. Sun Tzu, *The Art of War*, Samuel B. Griffith, trans. (New York: Oxford University Press, 1963), 84.
5. Leonard Caum Moffitt, *Global Positioning for the Twenty-First Century: Rethinking Strategic Planning* (East Lansing, MI: Michigan State University Press, 1990), 2.
6. John Lewis Gaddis, "Grand Strategy in the Second Term," *Foreign Affairs* 84, no. 1 (January 2005): 10.
7. X (George Kennan), "The Sources of Soviet Conduct," *Foreign Affairs* 25, no. 4 (July 1947): 566.
8. Kamran Taremi, "Iranian Strategic Culture: The Impact of Ayatollah Khomeini's Interpretation of Shiite Islam," *Contemporary Security Policy* 35, no. 1 (2014): 3–25.
9. Ahmad Nizar Hamzeh, *In the Path of Hizbullah* (Syracuse, NY: Syracuse University Press, 2004), 33–36. Also see Hezbollah Secretary General Hasan Nasrallah's views from one of his speeches at YouTube, September 19, 2014, https://www.youtube.com/watch?v=9chtFW4e2eg (accessed January 12, 2017).
10. David Commins, "Hasan al-Banna (1906–1949)," *Pioneers of Islamic Revival*, edited by Ali Rahnema, 2nd edition (London: Zed Books, 2006), 125–153.
11. Charles Tripp, "Sayyid Qutb," in Rahnema, *Pioneers of Islamic Revival*, 154–183.
12. Masoud Kazemzadeh, "Ayatollah Khamenei's Foreign Policy Orientation," *Comparative Strategy* 32, no. 5 (2013): 443–458; and Baqer Moin, "Khomeini's Search for Perfection," in Rahnema, *Pioneers of Islamic Revival*, 64–97.
13. Ariel Ahram, "Republic of Iraq," in *The Government and Politics of the Middle East and North Africa*, edited by Mark Gasiorowski and Sean L. Yom, 8th edition (Boulder, CO: Westview Press), 235–237.
14. Ibid., 237–239.
15. There were at least six major successful coups in 1936, 1958, February 8, 1963, November 1963, July 17, 1968, and July 1979. There have also been many unsuccessful coup attempts.
16. Ahram, 243.
17. Ibid., 253, 255.
18. Ofra Bingio, "With the Support of Iran Maliki Is Trying to Use the PUK and Goran to Divide Kurdish Camp and to Frustrate the Plan for Independence," interview with Gulan Media, November 14, 2016, http://gulan-media.com/english/details.php?section=2&id=166 (accessed August 1, 2017).
19. Masoud Kazemzadeh, "The Perils and Costs of a Grand Bargain with the Islamic Republic of Iran," *American Foreign Policy Interests*, 29, no. 5 (November 2007): 301–327.
20. Ahram, 242.
21. Ayatollah Ruhollah Khomeini, "Last Will and Testament," February 15, 1983, released after his death in June 1989, https://www.al-islam.org/imam-khomeini-s-last-will-and-testament (accessed June 15, 2017). The words within brackets are by the official translator, the words within {} are by me.
22. Alma Keshavarz, "Iran: al-Qaeda's 'Main Artery for Funds, Personnel and Communications': The Recently Released Osama bin Laden Letters," *Small Wars Journal*, March 10, 2016, http://smallwarsjournal.com/jrnl/art/iran-al-qaeda%E2%80%99s-%E2%80%9Cmain-artery-for-funds-personnel-and-communication%E2%80%9D-the-recently-released-o (accessed March 15, 2016).
23. Carlotta Gall, "In Afghanistan U.S. Exits, and Iran Comes In," *The New York Times*, August 5, 2017.
24. Ibid.
25. Masoud Kazemzadeh, "Foreign Policy Decision Making in Iran and the Nuclear Program," *Comparative Strategy* 36 (August 2017); Kazemzadeh, "Ayatollah Khamenei's Foreign Policy Orientation"; and Kevjn Lim, "National Security Decision-Making in Iran," *Comparative Strategy* 34, no. 2 (2015): 149–168.

26. "*Farmandeh Sepah: Helal Shia Dar Hal Shekl Giri Ast*," [IRGC Commander: The Shia Crescent is Being Formed], Jahan News, April 21, 2015, http://www.jahannews.com/analysis/421468/فرمانده-سپاه-هلال-شیعی-حال-شکل-گیری (accessed January 5, 2017) Jahan News is a hardline site close to the IRGC.
27. "*Tahlil Sokhanano Farmandeh Niroyeh Qods Sepah Ba Mozoeh Jahan Islam*" [Analysis of the Speech of the Commander of the Qods Force of the IRGC on the Subject of the Islamic World], Fars News Agency, March 29, 2014, http://www.farsnews.com/newstext.php?nn=13930108000154 (accessed January 5, 2017). My translation.
28. Ibid.
29. Ibid.
30. John Mearsheimer, "A Return to Offshore Balancing," *Newsweek*, December 30, 2008, http://www.newsweek.com/return-offshore-balancing-82925 (accessed October 10, 2015).
31. Hal Brands, *The Limits of Offshore Balancing* (U.S. Army War College, 2015), http://www.strategicstudiesinstitute.army.mil/pubs/display.cfm?pubID=1291 (accessed October 1, 2015). Christopher Layne, "America's Middle East Grand Strategy after Iraq: The Moment for Offshore Balancing Has Arrived," *Review of International Studies* 35, no. 1 (2009): 5–25.
32. David Remnick, "Going the Distance: On and Off the Road with Barack Obama," *The New Yorker*, January 27, 2014, http://www.newyorker.com/magazine/2014/01/27/going-the-distance-david-remnick (accessed August 5, 2016).
33. Jeffry Goldberg, "The Obama Doctrine," *The Atlantic*, April 2016, http://www.theatlantic.com/magazine/archive/2016/04/the-obama-doctrine/471525/ (accessed August 14, 2016).
34. "White House Rebuffed Clinton-Petraeus Plan to Arm Syrian Rebel: Report," Reuters, February 2, 2013, http://www.reuters.com/article/us-usa-syria-clinton-idUSBRE91201220130203 (accessed August 17, 2016).
35. Al Jazeera, "Counting the Cost, Iran's Rising Influence," March 28, 2015, YouTube, https://www.youtube.com/watch?v=-mKSycbUWn0 (accessed August 14, 2016).
36. Eli Lake, "Iran Spends Billions to Prop Up Assad," Bloomberg, June 9, 2015, https://www.bloomberg.com/view/articles/2015-06-09/iran-spends-billions-to-prop-up-assad (accessed June 15, 2017).
37. Lucas Tomlinson, "US Officials: Up to 100,000 Iranian-Backed Fighters Now in Iraq," Fox News, August 16, 2016, http://www.foxnews.com/politics/2016/08/16/us-officials-up-to-100000-iran-backed-fighters-now-in-iraq.html (accessed August 17, 2016).
38. Sebastian Maisel, "Kingdom of Saudi Arabia," in *The Government and Politics of the Middle East and North Africa*, edited by Gasiorowski and Yom, 319.
39. "Khobar Towers Press Release," FBI, Department of Justice, June 21, 2001, http://www.au.af.mil/au/awc/awcgate/khobar/khobar_fbi.htm (accessed October 10, 2015).
40. Eli Lake, "Why Obama Let Iran's Green Revolution Fail," Bloomberg, August 24, 2016, https://www.bloomberg.com/view/articles/2016-08-24/why-obama-let-iran-s-green-revolution-fail (accessed August 27, 2016).
41. Ibid.
42. Ibid.
43. Eli Lake and Josh Rogin, "Congress Alarmed by Iran Pact's Secret Understandings," Bloomberg, July 25, 2015, https://www.bloomberg.com/view/articles/2015-07-24/congress-alarmed-by-iran-pact-s-secret-understandings (accessed March 25, 2017).
44. Josh Meyer, "Obama's Hidden Iran Deal Giveaway," Politico, April 24, 2017, http://www.politico.com/story/2017/04/24/obama-iran-nuclear-deal-prisoner-release-236966 (accessed May 5, 2017).
45. Nasser Karimi, "Iran's FM Extolls Country's Ability to Restore Nuke Program," Associated Press, July 19, 2016, http://bigstory.ap.org/article/2f0bf5fb888348b3a274832a743dd521/irans-fm-extolls-countrys-ability-restore-nuke-program (accessed August 17, 2016).
46. George Jahn, "AP Exclusive: Document Shows Less Limit on Iran Nuke Work," Associated Press, July 18, 2016, http://www.bigstory.ap.org/article/140ca41aba7a42cda13792f07df4b8d3/ap-exclusive-secret-document-lifts-iran-nuke-constraints (accessed August 17, 2016).
47. Ambassador Stephen D. Mull, Lead Coordinator for Iran Nuclear Implementation, Senate Committee on Banking, House, and Urban Affairs, May 25, 2016, http://www.banking.senate.gov/public/_cache/files/6cec367e-fa69-4f0c-80d3-ed198084a5ce/C625C95FD44D63E153A005DABDAD88FF.052616-mull-testimony.pdf (accessed July 14, 2016).
48. Federal Ministry of the Interior, *2015 Annual Report on the Protection of the Constitution*, http://www.bmi.bund.de/SharedDocs/Downloads/EN/Broschueren/2016/vsb-kurzfassung-engl-2015.pdf?__blob=publicationFile (accessed July 14, 2016).
49. Polina Garaev, "Iran Still Trying to Acquire Materials for Nuclear Program, Germany Warns," i24 news, http://www.i24news.tv/en/news/international/119127-160707-iran-still-trying-to-acquire-materials-for-nuclear-program-germany-warns, July 7, 2016 (accessed July 14, 2016).
50. Ibid.
51. David Albright and Andrea Stricker, "Iranian Atomic Energy Organization Attempted Carbon Fiber Procurement," Institute for Science and International Security, July 7, 2016, http://isis-online.org/isis-reports/detail/iranian-atomic-energy-organization-attempted-carbon-fiber-procurement/ (accessed July 14 2016).

52. David Albright, Serena Kelleher-Vergantini, and Andrea Stricker, "Parchin: Will the IAEA Verify the Absence of Nuclear Weapons Activities in Iran?" Institute for Science and International Security, June 20, 2016, http://isis-online.org/uploads/isis-reports/documents/Parchin_Post_Implementation_Day_June_20_2016_Final.pdf (accessed July 14, 2016).
53. "State Department Spokesman Has Trouble Responding to German Intel Report about Iran," YouTube, July 8, 2016, https://www.youtube.com/watch?v=RhIO-ACGLMw (accessed July 14, 2016).
54. The previous six paragraphs are drawn, with minor changes, from Masoud Kazemzadeh, "Explaining The Obama Administration Overlooking Iran's Cheating on the Nuke Deal," *Small Wars Journal*, August 18, 2016, http://smallwarsjournal.com/blog/explaining-the-obama-administration-overlooking-iran%E2%80%99s-cheating-on-the-nuke-deal.
55. Donald Trump, "Transcript of President Trump's Speech in Riyadh," May 21, 2017, https://www.voanews.com/a/trump-speech-in-riyadh/3864144.html (accessed May 22, 2017).
56. Karen Parrish, "Mattis Meets with Saudi Officials in Riyadh, Praises Kingdom's Leadership," DOD News, April 19, 2017, https://www.defense.gov/News/Article/Article/1156947/ (accessed May 20, 2017).
57. Rex Tillerson, "Secretary of State Rex Tillerson Press Availability," April 19, 2017 https://www.state.gov/secretary/remarks/2017/04/270341.htm (accessed April 20, 2017).
58. For example, see "A Discussion on National Security with CIA Director Mike Pompeo," Center for Strategic & International Studies, April 13, 2017, https://www.csis.org/analysis/discussion-national-security-cia-director-mike-pompeo (accessed April 20, 2017).
59. Lesley Wroughton, "U.S. Says Iran Complies with Nuke Deal but Orders Review on Lifting Sanctions," Reuters, April 19, 2017, http://www.reuters.com/article/us-iran-nuclear-usa-tillerson-idUSKBN17L08I (accessed April 25, 2017).
60. CIA World Factbook, "Turkey," https://www.cia.gov/library/publications/the-world-factbook/geos/tu.html (accessed August 7, 2017).
61. Henri Barkey and Omer Taspinar, "Republic of Turkey," in *The Government and Politics of the Middle East and North Africa*, edited by Gasiorowski and Yom, 215.
62. CIA World Factbook, "Iran," https://www.cia.gov/library/publications/the-world-factbook/geos/ir.html (accessed August 7, 2017).
63. Thomas Sancton, "The Tehran Connection," *Time Magazine*, June 24, 2001, http://content.time.com/time/magazine/article/0,9171,164031,00.html (accessed January 20, 2017); Iran Human Rights Documentation Center, *No Safe Haven: Iran's Global Assassination Campaign*, May 2008, http://www.iranhrdc.org/english/publications/reports/3152-no-safe-haven-iran-s-global-assassination-campaign.html (accessed January 20, 2017).
64. Ibid.
65. United Nations, Commission on Human Rights, *Question of the Violation of Human Rights ...: Final Report on the Situation of Human Rights in the Islamic Republic of Iran Prepared by the Special Representative of the Commission on Human Rights, Mr. Reynaldo Galindo Pohl*, number E/CN.4/1994/50 (February 2, 1994), paragraph 209.
66. Benjamin Miller, "Explaining Changes in U.S. Grand Strategy: 9/11, the Rise of Offensive Liberalism, and the War in Iraq," *Security Studies* 19, no. 1 (2010): 26–65; David C. Ellis, "U.S. Grand Strategy Following the George W. Bush Presidency," *International Studies Perspectives* 10, no. 4 (2009): 361–377; and Heather S. Gregg, "Crafting a Better US Grand Strategy in the Post-September 11 World," *Foreign Policy Analysis* 6, no. 3 (July 2010): 237–255.
67. Gaddis, "Grand Strategy," 2–15.
68. Jeffry Goldberg, "The Obama Doctrine."
69. Hillary R. Clinton, "Hillary Clinton Addresses the Iran Nuclear Deal," The Brookings Institution, September 9, 2015, https://www.youtube.com/watch?v=eIqYRI1Fw2I (accessed August 24, 2016).
70. Julian Hattem, "Clinton Sides with Dem Leaders on Iran Sanctions," *The Hill*, September 1, 2016, http://thehill.com/policy/national-security/294164-clinton-sides-with-dem-leaders-on-iran-sanctions-ahead-of-standoff (accessed September 4, 2016).
71. Ibid.
72. James Traub, "The Hillary Clinton Doctrine," Foreign Policy, November 6, 2015, http://foreignpolicy.com/2015/11/06/hillary-clinton-doctrine-obama-interventionist-tough-minded-president/ (accessed July 7, 2016); and Perry Bacon, Jr., "How Hillary Clinton Would Differ from President Obama's Foreign Policy," NBC News, July 3, 2016, http://www.nbcnews.com/meet-the-press/how-hillary-clinton-would-alter-president-obama-s-foreign-policy-n589871 (accessed July 7, 2016).
73. Layne, "America's Middle East Grand Strategy."
74. Robert J. Lieber, "Staying Power and the American Future: Problems of Primacy, Policy, and Grand Strategy," *Journal of Strategic Studies* 34, no. 4 (August 2011): 509–530.

U.S.–Iran Confrontation in the Post-NIE World: An Analysis of Alternative Policy Options

MASOUD KAZEMZADEH

The United States, Israel, and several European allies have explicitly stated that they will not accept the possession of nuclear weapons by the Islamic fundamentalist regime ruling Iran. Iran has defied several UN Security Council resolutions and continued its uranium enrichment. On December 3, 2007, the U.S. released the November 2007 National Intelligence Estimate (NIE) on Iran. If the NIE assessment that Iran could develop nuclear weapons sometimes between 2010 and 2015 is correct, the new American president has twelve options available in dealing with Iran. This study analyzes potential consequences, shortcomings, costs, and benefits of each option.

The confrontation between the United States and Iran had escalated to new heights by late 2007. Defying two United Nations (UN) Security Council resolutions, Iran not only did not suspend its uranium enrichment process but succeeded in connecting about 3,000 centrifuges producing enriched uranium on a much larger scale. The United States, Israel, and several European allies explicitly stated that they would not accept the possession of nuclear bombs by the Islamic fundamentalist regime ruling Iran. Then, on December 3, 2007, the U.S. released the November 2007 National Intelligence Estimate (NIE) report entitled "Iran: Nuclear Intentions and Capabilities."[1] The NIE report made the surprising assessment that Iran halted its nuclear weapons program in 2003. The report further added that Iran would not be close to acquiring nuclear weapons until late 2009, but would probably have the capability to develop nuclear weapons sometime between 2010 and 2015.

The argument for military action was based on the perception that Iran was on the verge of acquiring nuclear weapons. The findings of the 2007 NIE undermined the urgency of surgical strikes in 2008 and early 2009. Because of this report, the Bush administration had extreme difficulty convincing others of the necessity of the military option in 2008. Moreover, China and Russia have referenced the NIE report to harden their opposition to tough UN Security Council sanctions on Iran. If the assessment that Iran could develop nuclear weapons sometime between 2010 and 2015 is correct, the Obama administration has twelve options available in dealing with Iran. This study analyzes potential consequences, shortcomings, costs, and benefits of each option.

Many Western leaders have been explicit in their insistence that due to the nature of the fundamentalist regime ruling Iran, they will not accept Iran developing nuclear weapons or having the capability of producing nuclear weapons. The threshold may not be the actual possession of nuclear weapons, but rather the mastery of the capability of producing nuclear weapons, such as enrichment of weapons grade uranium.[2] Iranian officials insist that Iran will continue its uranium enrichment, which would provide the regime the capability to produce nuclear weapons.

President Bush stated: "If you're interested in avoiding World War III, it seems like you ought to be interested in preventing them from having the knowledge necessary to make a nuclear weapon."[3] Four days later, Vice President Dick Cheney said: "Our country, and the international community, cannot stand by as a terror-supporting state fulfills its grandest ambitions . . . We will not allow Iran to have a nuclear weapon."[4] And that if Iran continues on its present course, the United States and other countries are "prepared to impose serious consequences."[5] Several days earlier, Admiral Michael Mullen, the Chairman of the Joint Chiefs of Staff, stated that military strikes are the last resort and the focus is currently on diplomacy, but if they fail to stop Iran's nuclear program, the United States has "more than enough reserves to respond" militarily.[6]

These words were accompanied by executive and legislative measures. On October 25, 2007, President Bush issued an executive order declaring the Qods Force of the Islamic Revolutionary Guards Corps (IRGC) a terrorist organization, adding names of individuals and IRGC companies to the list of terrorist entities, and directing the U.S. Treasury to convince various financial institutions around the world to freeze their accounts and stop any financial dealings with them.[7] A month earlier, on September 25, the U.S. House of Representatives passed the Iran Counter-Proliferation Act targeting IRGC's Qods Force with 397 votes for and 16 votes against. On September 26, in a nonbinding "sense of the Senate" resolution, the Senate passed an amendment to designate the Qods Force a terrorist organization. The amendment, named the Kyl-Lieberman amendment, passed 76 to 22 with 25 Democratic senators voting for it while two Republicans voted against it.

The Bush administration's determination to prevent the fundamentalist regime from acquiring nuclear weapons appears much stronger than many seem to appreciate. For example, the United States 2002 Nuclear Posture Review, which was leaked to the press, included potential nuclear strikes against Iran's nuclear facilities.[8] In the months after the 2007 NIE report was published, the Bush administration succeeded in getting the UN Security Council to pass a third resolution. Like the previous two, the third resolution was extremely mild, failing to induce Iran's leaders to change their policy.

Many Israelis appear to be convinced that if Iran were to possess nuclear weapons, these weapons would be used to wipe Israel off the map. Israeli officials have repeatedly stated that they regard nuclear weapons in the possession of the fundamentalist regime in Iran as an "existential threat" to Israel.[9] Perceptions of reality, whether true or false, many times determine behavior. And the perception of Israeli decisionmakers is that Iran is developing nuclear weaponry and will use it against them.[10] In a surprise trip to the Kremlin in late October 2007, Israel's Prime Minister, Ehud Olmert, reportedly told Russian President Vladimir Putin that Israel increasingly regards Iran as an Israeli problem that might require an Israeli military response, perhaps signaling his frustration with the lack of global response as well as Israeli determination to act unilaterally if Russia does not support Western powers in tough sanctions.[11] The Israeli government does not accept the judgments of the NIE report.[12] A recent study reports that, contrary to general perception, the Israeli air force has the capability to destroy Iran's most significant nuclear facilities in surgical air strikes.[13] In addition, Israel possesses submarines that could inflict serious damage to secondary facilities with submarine-launched cruise missiles.[14] In no uncertain term, Israeli officials have indicated that they will use military strikes to attack Iran's nuclear facilities. For example, in early June 2008, Israel carried out major military exercises whose purpose was widely regarded to convey its seriousness to attack Iranian nuclear facilities.[15]

French President Nicolas Sarkozy, in August 2007, pushed for serious sanctions in order to avoid "a catastrophic alternative: an Iranian bomb, or the bombing of Iran."[16] The French strong position comes as a surprise considering its huge economic relations with Iran. French lenders hold some $5.9 billion, the largest of any in the European Union (EU), and some French companies, such as auto maker Renault and oil company Total SA, are major players in the Iranian economy.[17] Sarkozy has been explicitly advocating negotiation with Iran in order to convince Iranian officials to stop their nuclear program, while holding the use of military attack as the last option to be used if Iran refuses.

By mid-2008, officials in the United States, the United Kingdom, France, and Israel had explicitly stated that the military option is available to prevent Iran from developing nuclear weapons and/or the capability to develop nuclear weapons. Other great powers such as Germany, China, and Russia have stated that they oppose the development of nuclear weapons and uranium enrichment by Iran, but they have not placed the military option on the table and insist that diplomacy can convince Iranian officials to stop their nuclear activities.

Iranian officials, including Supreme Leader Ali Khamenei and President Mahmoud Ahmadinejad, have explicitly and publicly stated that they will proceed with the enrichment process. They claim that Iran's nuclear program is solely for peaceful purposes. Several UN Security Council resolutions had failed to convince Iran's leaders to stop their nuclear-related activities such as uranium enrichment. President Ahmadinejad has repeatedly dismissed repeated warnings of American military strikes against nuclear facilities as empty rhetoric. Ahmadinejad argued that there was no possibility of American military conflict because "American policies in the region have met with defeat and they are forced to leave the region in the near future."[18]

Ahmadinejad has succeeded in removing officials who are not as extremist as he is and replacing them with individuals who share his extremist policies. This indicates a purge of individuals who advocate policies based on negotiations with those more willing to take a much harder line on nuclear issues, such as no suspension of uranium enrichment.

If Iran is not willing to give up its nuclear enrichment process, there are twelve primary options available to the United States and the international community. Several options may be combined sequentially or simultaneously, and one option may also quickly give way to another. The twelve primary options are:

- Option 1: Military action (surgical strikes)
- Option 2: Military action (massive prolonged strikes)
- Option 3: Military action (regime change via military action and occupation; Iraq and Afghanistan models)
- Option 4: Military action (ground invasion, discovery and destruction of nuclear facilities, leave and see what happens; possible disintegration of Iran)
- Option 5: Dialogue (limited issue-based dialogue; North Korean model)
- Option 6: Grand bargain (Libyan model)
- Option 7: Do nothing (and perhaps acquiesce to a nuclear weapons capability)
- Option 8: UN Security Council comprehensive sanctions
- Option 9: Reconfigured containment
- Option 10: Naval blockade
- Option 11: Covert operations
- Option 12: Regime change via nonviolent struggle

Military Options

Proponents of the military options argue that due to the extremist, fanatical, and terrorist nature of the regime ruling Iran, its possession of nuclear weapons would undermine world peace and security. In addition, deterrence may not work due to the central role of *shehadat-talabi* (martyrdom-seeking) in Shia belief system. The rise to prominence by the apocalyptic elements in Iran and the repeated public pronouncement of Iran's president about the destruction of Israel have given rise to great urgency and worry in many capitals, including but not limited to Washington and Tel Aviv. Therefore, many have declared that one could not live with this regime possessing nuclear weapons or the capability to produce such weapons.

Many scholars have demonstrated that deterrence between fully rational actors during the Cold War had many near failures and that one could not rely upon deterrence in the post-Cold War period, especially with leaders with apocalyptic and martyrdom-seeking belief systems.[19] If one accepts that the Shia fundamentalist leaders of Iran cannot be deterred, and one assumes that Iran is pursuing a clandestine nuclear weapons program, then the only way to stop Iran from possessing such weapons is to destroy its nuclear facilities. There are four major military options.

Option 1: Military Action (Surgical Strikes)

Some support the view that only surgical strikes are necessary. The primary goal is to destroy the main nuclear facilities, which would destroy, or at least postpone, Iran's capability to develop nuclear weapons. The most detailed public discussion of this position was presented by Norman Podhoretz, a principal foreign policy advisor to Rudy Giuliani.[20] Another policymaker, Joshua Muravchik, a member of the State Department's Advisory Committee on Democracy Promotion, writes: "Our choice is stark. Accept Iran with an atom bomb or cripple its nuclear program by force. Nothing will stop Tehran . . . Only strikes against Iran's nuclear facilities can forestall these terrible scenarios . . . We would send no troops, conquer no land. Rather, we would act in pre-emptive self-defense."[21]

Both Podhoretz and Muravchik advocate surgical strikes. They argue that sanctions would have little or no effect in influencing Iran's rulers and the possibility of such sanctions spurring an uprising is unrealistic. Moreover, Russia and China would not vote for such comprehensive sanctions. Thus, the only way to stop Iran's nuclear weapons program is surgical strikes.

There are several serious problems with surgical strikes of nuclear facilities. First, there are many sites that are not known to the United States. Second, the Iranian regime possesses great retaliatory capabilities, including attacking oil shipments in the Persian Gulf and through the Strait of Hormuz,[22] attacking oil facilities of Western allies in the regions (Saudi Arabia, Kuwait, Qatar, UAE), unleashing its allies (Lebanese Hezbollah, Hamas, Palestinian Islamic Jihad) on Western interests, attacking American military personnel in the region (Iraq, Afghanistan, Bahrain, Qatar) directly or via proxies, and carrying out terrorist operations inside the United States with agents, sleeper cells, or proxies. At the very least, the Iranian regime seems capable of increasing American casualties in Iraq and hitting some oil tankers in the Persian Gulf. The fear of massive and effective retaliation by Iran would make surgical strikes less attractive than major and prolonged military operations aiming at regime change, which is Option 2. Third, surgical strikes (in contradistinction to massive strikes targeting coercive apparatuses of the regime such as IRGC, Basij paramilitary forces, and the Ministry of Intelligence, as advocated by Option 2), which would leave the coercive apparatuses intact, would actually increase the hold of the hard-line elements over the entire society, which would take advantage of the situation and utterly silence the little space that exists in civil society.

Option 1 would only make sense if one assumes that Iran would not retaliate. In all likelihood, the fundamentalist regime would retaliate, as has been repeated by numerous officials. Supreme Leader Ali Khamenei warned, "The Americans should know that if they assault Iran, their interests will be harmed anywhere in the world that is possible . . . The

Iranian nation will respond to any blow with double the intensity."[23] In the words of Iran's Defense Minister, Brig. Gen. Mostafa Mohammad Najar: "With determination and using all the options—without limit in time and space—we will give a destructive response to any hostile action."[24] One might dismiss Iran's consistent threats of retaliation as a bluff. From the Iranian perspective, however, a massive retaliation might be their best choice. If Iran did not retaliate, and instead simply accelerated their nuclear program, the United States would repeat surgical strikes again and again. Nuclear facilities are terribly expensive for Iran, but the costs of missiles are insignificant for Americans. Iranian leaders realize that not retaliating in a total and prohibitive manner would create a losing dynamic for Iran. From Iranian leaders' point of view, the worst situation would be the utterly humiliating and costly option of having their nuclear facilities repeatedly destroyed without any response. Not having a nuclear program would be more preferable than having them destroyed by recurring American surgical strikes. Iran's leaders assume that the United States does not have enough boots needed for an invasion because their forces are bogged down in Iraq and Afghanistan; therefore, a massive retaliation would cause American retreat. The costs to Iran would be acceptable, but more significantly, an American defeat would propel Iran to the status of the regional hegemon with unlimited benefits.

The Iranian government would try to close off the Strait of Hormuz, through which a large portion of the internationally traded oil passes. If the Iranian government is able to keep the Strait closed for several months, it could cause a collapse of the global economy. If it could close the Strait for a few weeks, then it would cause much economic harm. The worst-case scenario would include successful closure of the Strait, mass attacks on American targets in Iraq and Afghanistan,[25] attacks on U.S.-friendly governments in Saudi Arabia, Kuwait, Qatar, Bahrain, UAE, Turkey, Pakistan, Lebanon, and Israel, and terrorist attacks against civilians in Western Europe and in the United States.

Option 2: Military Action (Massive Prolonged Strikes)

Concerned about retaliation, others advocate massive attacks on coercive and political targets in addition to nuclear facilities with the goals of not only destroying nuclear capabilities but also undermining retaliatory capabilities. There is also the hope of causing mass uprising, leading to the overthrow of the regime.

From the perspective of the proponents of Option 2, the best-case scenario is that the overwhelming majority of Iranians would either support the U.S. military action or remain neutral, as many Kurds did during the U.S. invasion of Iraq in 2003. Would Iranians behave as did the Iraqi Kurds (strong support), or the Iraqi Shia (mixed), or the Iraqi Sunni Arabs (strong opposition)? Would Iranian-armed opposition groups (Democratic Party of Iranian Kurdistan, Komala, PMOI, etc.) behave as did the Northern Alliance in Afghanistan? Would post-fundamentalist Iran become a democracy as did Germany, Italy, and Japan after WWII and Haiti and Bosnia and Herzegovina in the post-Cold War period, or would it look like Afghanistan and Iraq?

How would the Iranian people react to American bombings, which would destroy fundamentalist coercive apparatuses that have been brutalizing them? The honest answer is that we do not know what the reaction of the Iranian people would be. Would those so brutalized and oppressed for thirty years take advantage and take revenge on their oppressors? Or would they "rally around the flag" and help the fundamentalists to continue to rule them? Would Iranians, by and large, behave like the Kurds or Sunni Arabs or Shiite Arabs in Iraq? I surmise that some (mostly fundamentalists) would engage in fights against

Americans, while some would take advantage of the situation and attack the fundamentalists; and while some would sit on the sidelines cheering, others would sit on the sidelines fuming. What proportion of the population would be in each category cannot be known in advance. Those who confidently and categorically state what the Iranian people will do are probably projecting their own wishes. At best, we could surmise which action by each actor (e.g., U.S. government, fundamentalist regime, opposition groups) might increase or decrease the likelihood of proportions in each category.

Although massive American military strikes on coercive apparatuses of the regime may result in mass uprising leading to the overthrow of the regime, it is also likely that the war may lead to much chaos and/or disintegration of Iran into several mini-states. The likelihood of the latter scenarios increases if the regime does not fall immediately and if American strikes are accompanied with assistance to Iranian armed opposition forces (e.g., PMOI, Democratic Party of Iranian Kurdistan, Komala, and Balochi resistence groups, among others) willing to cooperate with the American invasion.

In early 2003, witnessing the swift crushing of the Taliban–al Qaeda regime in Afghanistan and Saddam's regime in Iraq, many Iranians publicly supported American military intervention in order to be "liberated from the yoke of the fundamentalist regime's dictatorship" as many put it.[26] Khomeini's grandson, Hojatolislam Seyyed Hussein Khomeini, publicly embraced an American invasion to liberate Iran from the dictatorial regime that his grandfather had created. Introduced by Michael Ledeen, Hussein Khomeini repeated his earlier remarks at an American Enterprise Institute conference. Representatives of the Democratic Party of Iranian Kurdistan met with Pentagon officials in May 2003. One of Iran's most respected Marxist intellectuals, Professor Kambiz Roosta, has publicly stated that due to the nature and bellicose policies of the fundamentalist regime, the United States has the right to use military force to overthrow it. The largest left-wing guerrilla group, the PMOI, closely cooperates with the U.S. (as it did with Saddam Hussein) against the fundamentalist regime. The U.S. forces in Iraq also have a policy of benign neglect toward Komala, a major Marxist Kurdish guerrilla organization, which regularly carries out crossborder military operations against the coercive apparatuses of the regime. Many conservative monarchists also support American military intervention to topple the fundamentalist regime. The most sophisticated is Dr. Sohrab Rob Sobhani, a close friend and advisor to Reza Pahlavi, who wishes to restore the Pahlavi monarchy.[27]

The horrific carnage in Iraq and the resilience of the Taliban in Afghanistan have caused many Iranians to have second thoughts about the potential benefits and costs of an American military invasion. Karim Sadjadpour, an astute observer of Iran who is an associate at the Carnegie Endowment for International Peace, has noted that unlike in 2003, many Iranians today prefer stability and tyranny to chaos and democracy.[28] Sadjadpour may be right or he may be wrong. It is quite possible that those who still wish for an American invasion to be freed from fundamentalist tyranny may still constitute a majority, but a silent majority. In mid-2008, another astute observer of Iran, Azadeh Moaveni, reported a new upsurge of support for American intervention in Iran, which she attributed to increased repression and the deteriorating economy under Ahmadinejad.[29]

Iranian officials seem to be genuinely worried about this scenario, which has a high likelihood of success in toppling the regime.[30] Much of the regime's propaganda assets are geared toward raising opposition around the world to this option by portraying the fundamentalist regime as an innocent victim of American and Israeli warmongers who wish to attack Iran for the purposes of controlling Middle Eastern oil and imposing American domination and imperialism around the globe.

Option 3: Military Action (Regime Change via Military Action and Occupation; Iraq and Afghanistan Models)

This option advocates a massive invasion leading to regime change. This option is based on the assumption that despite prolonged massive bombing, the fundamentalist regime would survive and could then carry out massive retaliation, thus necessitating a robust and quick American ground invasion to make certain that the regime is toppled before it could retaliate.

A major disadvantage with military actions that would not result in immediate overthrow of the regime is the potential disruption to oil supplies. If Iran is able to close off the Strait of Hormuz, that would bring catastrophic damage to the world economy. According to U.S. government data, in 2006, "the Persian Gulf countries . . . produced about 28 percent of the world's oil, while holding 55 percent (728 billion barrels) of the world's crude oil reserves. In 2006, the Persian Gulf countries combined exported 18.2 million barrels per day (bbl/d), including about 17 million bbl/d via the Strait of Hormuz, representing roughly one-fifth of the world oil supply."[31] In other words, about 20 percent of the world's oil supplies pass through the Strait of Hormuz. This is about 40 percent of the world's oil exports (internationally traded oil).[32]

If the United States is able to keep the Strait open and only block Iran's oil exports, then not much harm will come to the world economy. Since 1987, the U.S. Navy has been concerned about this issue, so it is presumed that the Navy has developed plans for this contingency. Iran exports 2.5 million barrels per day. Saudi Arabia produces about 8.7 million barrels per day and has the ability to boost output with another 2.5 million barrels per day, thus making up for the loss of Iranian oil.[33] Moreover, most industrialized countries have Strategic Petroleum Reserves (SPR) that can be used during emergencies. The United States SPR, for example, has almost 700 million barrels, which is equivalent to about 68 days of U.S. oil imports from all sources.[34] In 2006, the SPR of the United States and other members of the International Energy Agency was around 1.48 billion barrels.[35] If Iran succeeded in closing off the Strait, the United States would have somewhere between two and five months to either change the regime in Iran or concede defeat and leave the Persian Gulf area. Increased strategic reserves around the world would increase the time available to the United States to continue its operations. The two crucial battlegrounds will be the control of the Strait of Hormuz and the streets of Tehran.

Option 4: Military Action (Ground Invasion, Discovery and Destruction of Nuclear Facilities, Leave and See What Happens; Possible Disintegration of Iran)

This option argues that the costs of occupation might be high; therefore, after a massive invasion and overthrow of the fundamentalist regime, the American forces should concentrate on finding and destroying nuclear facilities. The U.S. forces would then evacuate and see what happens afterwards. The United States could live with the disintegration of Iran into several smaller countries. Such an option was not realistic in Afghanistan and Iraq, but it is realistic for Iran. The United States needed to occupy Afghanistan in order to prevent Taliban and al Qaeda return, which would enable them to plan and carry out terrorist activities against American interests. In Iraq, this was not desirable because the most likely outcome would have been ethno-sectarian civil war and the disintegration of Iraq into ethno-sectarian regions, thus inviting military interventions by Turkey, Iran, and possibly Saudi Arabia, Jordan, and Egypt. All of Iraq's neighbors intensely feared and strongly opposed disintegration of Iraq. Such concerns are absent for the case of Iran. On the contrary, Iran's neighbors, by and large, would be happy to see the disintegration of Iran.

The American military possesses great capabilities to quickly overthrow a regime, but it is ill-equipped to create a stable regime afterward, as demonstrated in Afghanistan and Iraq. Unlike the Taliban's regime and Saddam's regime, which were based on particular ethno-sectarian groups, the fundamentalist regime in Iran is not based on any ethnic group. Rather it is composed of supporters of an ideology, Shia fundamentalism. In Iran, not only do Sunni Kurds and Sunni Balochis intensely oppose the regime but, more significantly, the majority of Shia Persians, Azeris, Gilaks, and Mazandaranis do as well. Therefore, once overthrown, the fundamentalists lack a safe haven to regroup, resist, and struggle to come back to power. The Pashtun areas in Afghanistan and Pakistan, and Sunni Arab regions in Iraq provided such safe havens for Taliban and Saddam supporters. In other words, while it is extremely hard for the Iranian people to overthrow the fundamentalist regime, once overthrown, it would be very easy to keep the fundamentalists subdued. Leaving a country just after successfully invading it is counterintuitive and has little historical precedent. However, it is an option that appears to contain high benefits at relatively low costs.

Diplomacy

Proponents of this option believe that it might be possible to provide incentives (financial, political, and security) to the fundamentalist regime in exchange for the regime giving up its nuclear program that might give it nuclear weapons capability. Many skeptics of the ultimate utility of diplomacy argue that, before any resort to military options, the diplomatic route is necessary in order to illustrate that it is the Iranian government that refuses to give up nuclear weapons capability.[36] There are two suboptions: limited issue-based dialogue, and grand bargain.

Option 5: Limited Issue-Based Dialogue

Proponents of this policy believe that there is no serious nuclear threat from the Iranian regime and that much of the conflict is due to misunderstandings and misperceptions. Advocates of this option argue that Iranian leadership is rational and its primary objective is hegemony in its region, which has brought it into conflict with the United States. In order to prevent any unnecessary military engagement, it is necessary to reduce tensions between Iran and the United States. The United States should accede to Iran's legitimate interests in this region.[37] Due to the past thirty years of hostility, the United States should hold meetings on various issues of concern between the two countries with the goal of reaching agreements on the easiest issues first. Such agreements would reduce tensions and build trust between the two governments.

If Iran does not have a clandestine nuclear weapons program and its main goal is regional hegemony, then the best policy for the United States would be conventional containment or a reconfigured containment (see Option 9). Considering the unpopularity of the regime, the possibility of a transition to democracy in the medium term (e.g., the next ten years or so), and the high costs of military action, it would be best to avoid major military confrontation.

Option 6: Grand Bargain

Proponents of this policy argue that due to mutual distrust between the two governments, it would not be possible to reach meaningful agreements on any major issue because each would be very reluctant to give in on any issue to what it perceives to be its erstwhile enemy.[38] For example, if Iranian leadership believes that the United States intends to overthrow it, any assistance to Americans in stabilizing Iraq would free them to carry out their attacks on Iran soon after. Therefore, the only way to resolve the conflict is to put all the major issues on the table, where one side would be willing to give in on an issue of lesser significance to it while the other side would be willing to give in on another issue which holds a different degree of significance. For example, if Iranian leaders were assured that the United States would not pursue any policies that would threaten their survival, then they might be willing to help the United States stabilize Iraq. If the U.S. were provided assurances that Iran does not plan to develop nuclear weapons (by fully giving up all worrisome programs, such as uranium enrichment, under full IAEA inspections), then the United States could provide security assurances (i.e., no forced regime change) in return.

Diplomatic Pitfalls

If Iran does not have a clandestine nuclear weapons program, it would be to the benefit of the Iranian government to get all the concessions possible in exchange for something it does not have, but others believe it does. However, if the regime does have a clandestine nuclear weapons program, it would be against its interests to give that up. Unlike North Korea, which is desperately poor, Iran is incredibly rich in natural resources from oil to natural gas to copper. Therefore, tens of billions of dollars would not be an attractive incentive compared to the possession of nuclear weapons, if the possession of such weapons would accrue great-power status leading to the domination of the region, which itself is incredibly rich in natural resources.

If Iran's fundamentalist rulers truly wish to implement their ideology and ideals and export their revolution and become the regional hegemon, then they need nuclear weapons to succeed. Negotiation would not be of benefit to Iran's rulers if that meant actually giving up the putative clandestine nuclear weapons program. Negotiation would have only two benefits for Iran's rulers. First, it would buy time to complete the nuclear program. And second, it would provide status and prestige to compel the world's great powers to recognize them and give in to some of their demands.

The proposal for direct, unconditional negotiations may have several disadvantages. First, if such high-level direct and comprehensive negotiations were held and failed, then the United States would have to either publicly acquiesce to Iran's nuclear program or immediately use military attacks. The advantage of no direct and comprehensive negotiations is that it prevents the stark and immediate choice and allows more time to decide what to do, and when. In other words, if the United States were to engage in comprehensive high-level negotiations, and failed, then not only is the likelihood of war dramatically increased, but also at a time that is dictated by Iranian leaders. If the United States did not engage in direct comprehensive negotiations, it could use other means (e.g., global sanctions) and postpone any serious military confrontation until the time and manner of its choosing. The only advantage of direct comprehensive negotiation for the United States is its failure would bring many other powers to the side of the United States.

Second, because Iranian officials have a long and proven history of lying to the international community and deceptions, one could not trust that they would abide by the agreement or that they would disclose their clandestine nuclear program. If Iranian officials signed an agreement and did not reveal their clandestine nuclear program, either they would succeed in completing their nuclear weapons program or their deception would be discovered. In either case, the ramifications would be more grievous than not having had the failed agreement.

The lack of honesty is crucial here. Iranian officials kept their nuclear program hidden for more than eighteen years when it was exposed by an opposition group (PMOI). Furthermore, in October 2003, Iranian officials made a decision to lie to the EU-3 (Britain, France, and Germany), even after they promised they would disclose all the previous activities. According to Iran's then-top nuclear negotiator, Hojatolislam Hassan Rouhani, telling the Europeans the truth would have sent Iran's dossier to the UN Security Council; therefore, a decision was made at the highest levels of the regime to lie to the EU-3.[39] The regime was not aware that the Libyan government had disclosed all its nuclear programs to the United States and Britain. Thus, the Iranian regime decided not to reveal that it had secretly purchased the highly sophisticated P2 centrifuge plans. Because of the Libyan disclosures, though, the EU-3 and the IAEA were aware of the network that sold P2 centrifuge plans to Iran. Rouhani states that exposure of Iran's explicit deceptions caused the EU-3 to mistrust Iran. This caused the EU to support the American policy of referring Iran to the UN Security Council. Previously, the EU had been trying to undermine the American policy of referring Iran to the UN Security Council.

It is imperative to add that deceptions on Iran's nuclear file are not exceptions in the behavior of Iranian officials. The regime has a long history of explicit lies to promote its interests. For example, before gaining power, Khomeini explicitly promised freedom (even for Marxists) and democracy. Moreover, Khomeini repeatedly promised that he would not hold any position of power. But after consolidating power, Khomeini engaged in severe repression of dissidents, including high-ranking Shia clerics who opposed fundamentalists. Instead of democracy, Khomeini established an incredibly brutal dictatorship. Khomeini, of course, became the Supreme Leader, amassing executive, legislative, and judicial powers in his own hands.[40]

Fundamentalists justify such explicit lies as *maslehat* (expediency, interest) which are necessary to serve the *nizam* (system). Other examples of expedient dissimulation include the officials' public denials of the assassinations of dissidents abroad, despite the fact that the regime's agents had been arrested, convicted, and imprisoned in many Western European countries. Although the regime has successfully lobbied for the extradition of the imprisoned assassins to Iran, it denies that those agents were sent by the regime.[41] Another example of such deception is the regime officials promising dialogue with the secretary-general of the Democratic Party of Iranian Kurdistan to lure him into negotiations, only to assassinate him and two of his lieutenants during the negotiations in Vienna on July 13, 1989. Referring to fundamentalist officials, a Western diplomat serving in Tehran said, "Iran says the opposite of what it thinks and does the opposite of what it says, which does not necessarily mean that it does the opposite of what it thinks."[42]

Third, Iranian people are the most pro-American population in the Islamic world. The main reason is their perception that unlike other countries, the United States has taken their side against their oppressive government. By sitting down and reaching an agreement with the regime, Iranians who oppose the regime would feel betrayed and their positive sentiments toward the United States would dissipate. If, in fact, the regime has no clandestine nuclear weapons program, the United States would lose its popularity among Iranian people by making agreements with their unpopular leaders.

Negotiations would be in the American national interest, however, if Iran does have a clandestine nuclear weapons program and negotiations could cause Iran's fundamentalist leaders to honestly declare and dismantle them. Negotiations would also be in American interests if Iran does have a clandestine nuclear weapons program and is willing to publicly declare it (but not dismantle it) and one assumes that deterrence would work (as did detente with the former USSR and China).

Option 7: Do Nothing (and Perhaps Acquiesce to a Nuclear Weapons Capability)

Proponents of this option argue that a nuclear Iran is inevitable, deterrence works, there is no military option, and the world must learn to live with a nuclear Iran, including recognizing Iran's ambitions to be the hegemonic power in the region. The so-called "do nothing" option believes that giving in to Iran's demands would not cause a major threat to the international order, peace, and stability; that Iranian rulers are fully rational; and that conventional deterrence would work in deterring them from the use of their nuclear weapons in a first strike on Israel.

The most sophisticated proponent of this position is Kenneth Waltz, who argues that Iran's leaders are rational, that it is in their interests to develop nuclear weapons, and they could be deterred just like Stalin's USSR and Mao's China were.[43] Waltz believes in the realist assumption that domestic policies of other states have little or no bearing on their foreign policies, that all states are rational, that they could be deterred by America's nuclear arsenal, and that foreign policy should not be influenced by notions of human rights, democracy, and freedom that animates their old paradigmatic rival, the idealists, and their current nemesis, the neoconservatives. Waltz argues that he has observed nothing that would indicate Iran's leaders are irrational, thus making an exception to realist assumption. Moreover, getting nuclear weapons by Iran's leaders is rational because those weapons would serve as a deterrent against American invasion and regime change.[44]

The best-case scenario in the "do nothing" option is that the fundamentalist regime would not develop nuclear weapons. Lesser good scenarios would be that if the fundamentalist regime did, in fact, acquire nuclear weapons, it would not drop them on Israel, or give them to its terrorist proxies, or use them to threaten others in order to impose its hegemony.[45]

The worst-case scenario in the "do nothing" option includes an Iranian preemptive nuclear strike against Israel. This would result in an American or Israeli nuclear retaliation, causing tens of millions of Iranian deaths. The worst-case scenario may cause the deaths of up to 70 million Iranians and up to 11 million in Israel/Palestine (about seven million Jews and four million Palestinians who live between the Mediterranean sea and the River Jordan).[46] Considering the prevalence of apocalyptic ideology (i.e., the 12th Imam) and the Shiite belief in the desirability of mass martyrdom (i.e., the 3rd Imam's mass martyrdom in Karbala) among Ahmadinejad's inner circle, a preemptive nuclear strike may not be as out of the question as one could logically posit among Marxist-Leninist regimes in the former Soviet Union and China.[47]

Another bad scenario in the "do nothing" option would be if Iran used its nuclear weapons as a shield against any American military attack in order to massively intervene in Iraq to push the United States out. If this were to occur, then the question would be whether the United States would enter a war with Iran or leave Iraq. And if the United States were to leave Iraq, would other regional states acquiesce or would they enter the war against Iran in Iraq? Would Iran resort to nuclear bombs if it were to lose a war against other regional powers (e.g., a coalition of Sunni states)? Would Pakistan come to the assistance of fellow Sunnis or would it stay out? Would the Iranian regime invade Bahrain, Kuwait, Qatar, or the UAE? Would the Shiites in the oil-rich eastern province of Saudi Arabia rise up against the Wahhabi state and request assistance from the Shiite regime in Iran? Would Iran invade Saudi Arabia to liberate fellow Shiites?

What precisely does hegemony mean in this context? Would Khamenei and Ahmadinejad follow the letter of Iran's 1979 constitution and export their revolution and fulfill Khomeini's dream, or would they betray their own ideals and constitution?

The constitution created by the fundamentalists in 1979 states:

> With due attention to the Islamic content of the Iranian Revolution, the Constitution provides the necessary basis for ensuring the continuation of the Revolution at home and abroad. In particular, in the development of international relations, the Constitution will strive with other Islamic and popular movements to prepare the way for the formation of a single world community (in accordance with the Koranic verse "This your community is a single community, and I am your Lord, so worship Me" [21:92]), and to assure the continuation of the struggle for the liberation of all deprived and oppressed peoples in the world . . . .
>
> *An Ideological Army*
>
> In the formation and equipping of the country's defence forces, due attention must be paid to faith and ideology as the basic criteria. Accordingly, the Army of the Islamic Republic of Iran and the Islamic Revolutionary Guards Corps are to be organized in conformity with this goal, and they will be responsible not only for guarding and preserving the frontiers of the country, but also for fulfilling the ideological mission of jihad in God's way; that is, extending the sovereignty of God's law throughout the world (this is in accordance with the Koranic verse "Prepare against them whatever force you are able to muster, and strings of horses, striking fear into the enemy of God and your enemy, and others besides them" [8:60]).[48]

The main slogans of the regime, which express their ideals, have been: *Marg bar America* (Death to America) and *Marg bar Israel* (Death to Israel). Would the fundamentalist leaders use nuclear weapons to implement their slogans? Should one dismiss such slogans as meaningless rhetoric or recognize them as a reflection of the true ideals of true believers? In other words, based on observations of the behavior of Iran's leaders since 1978–79, can one discern a pattern of a predilection for rhetoric without action or a patter of predilection to implement their words into action?

In the past thirty years, the fundamentalists have tried to implement their slogans with actual violent actions. Taking over the U.S. Embassy and holding Americans hostage for 444 days was not mere rhetoric but constituted an attack on the sovereign territory of another nation. After the liberation of the Iranian city, Khorramshahr, in 1982, Iraqi forces were almost completely out of Iranian territories. Saddam Hussein called for ceasefire and official cessation of hostilities. To encourage Ayatollah Khomeini to accept the ceasefire, Saudi Arabia and other Arab states offered Iran huge sums for reparations. After a lull of few months in actual warfare, Khomeini and his lieutenants decided to carry the war into Iraqi territory. They initially demanded Saddam's resignation, and when Iran crossed into Iraqi territory, the main slogan was *Rah-e Qods az Karbala Migozarad* (the Road to

Jerusalem Passes Through Karbala). To emphasize the main goal of the war, most of the major campaigns into Iraq were named *Qods* 1 (Jerusalem 1), *Qods* 2 (Jerusalem 2) and the like. Whereas Saddam portrayed the eight-year war to be a war between Arabs and Persians, the rulers of Iran portrayed the war as war between the forces of Islam against the forces of American imperialism, Israeli Zionism, and their local Arab lackeys. What is instructive is that while Iranian officials declared Saddam to be a Zionist and an American stooge, they engaged in secret negotiations with American officials and Israelis to get weapons in what became known as the Iran-Contra scandal. Iranian officials' condemnation of various regimes in the region has not been limited to empty rhetoric. The governments of Egypt, Saudi Arabia, Algeria, and Bahrain have accused the fundamentalist regime of clandestinely assisting extremist terrorist groups in attempts to overthrow their governments.[49]

Another bad scenario of the "do nothing" option would be if Iran were to use its nuclear weapons as a shield to massively increase assistance to the Lebanese Hezbollah and Syria in order to create a Shiite fundamentalist regime in Lebanon and subjugate non-Shiite groups in Lebanon. With nuclear weapons, Iran would feel free to spread its control in the region directly and/or through proxies.

If Iran gains nuclear weapons, there is an incentive for other powers in the region such as Saudi Arabia, Egypt, and Turkey to gain nuclear weapons of their own. Considering the weaknesses of these states, the possibilities of terrorists gaining these weapons through theft or surreptitious transfer and possessing them after the collapse of the state is likely.

Coercive Diplomacy

Option 8: UN Security Council Comprehensive Sanctions

Proponents of this option argue that the imposition of serious universal sanctions on the regime has the possibility of either producing a major change in the behavior of the regime or seriously undermining the regime, with the likelihood of enabling the Iranian people themselves to overthrow the regime. The advocates of this option argue that because it is possible, if not very likely, to get one of the truly horrific scenarios under earlier options, one should implement Option 8 before proceeding towards other options.

Because of the great costs, especially if the worst-case scenarios within each option were to occur, the comprehensive economic sanctions should be implemented before one tries either military options or appeasement. The best-case scenario under Option 8 would be a regime change. And the worst-case scenario would be buying time and postponing of the costly war or appeasing. This option would be most effective if the sanctions are global, that is, other great powers such as the EU, Russia, and China would participate. Although the proposal that EU, Japan, and other countries join the U.S. in imposing economic sanctions would have some effect, only a UN Security Council comprehensive sanction has real impact.

This option's best-case scenario of regime change before the acquisition of nuclear weapons (or know-how) would preclude the immediate necessity of both war and appeasement. Despite public demands that the international community, especially the EU, Russia, and China give serious consideration to this option, many of the principal actors have refrained from serious action.

This option has the lowest costs and the highest benefits to the international community (including Iranian people who oppose the regime). The costs involved are the loss of lucrative trade and the loss of oil contracts. These pale in comparison with the costs in human lives and economic catastrophe in the other options, so that it would be a reasonable sacrifice to prevent the much graver costs of other options.

The NIE report made it politically much harder for the Bush administration to convince China and Russia to support tough sanctions in late 2007 and 2008. However, one might argue that the Obama administration could make a powerful argument in 2009 that the NIE report makes a very strong case for sanctions for five reasons. First, the report is highly confident that despite its denials, Iran's government and military did have a nuclear weapons program. Second, although it halted this program in 2003, at a minimum it is keeping open its option to develop nuclear weapons. Third, Iran has advanced its civilian and dual-use nuclear technological infrastructure. Fourth, Tehran halted its nuclear weapons program in response to international scrutiny and pressure, suggesting that the regime does, in fact, respond to international pressure. Therefore, one may logically conclude that if pressures are removed, the regime would reconstitute its nuclear weapons program. Moreover, increased pressure may succeed in convincing Iran to abandon its enrichment process. Fifth, if Russia and China refused to support sanctions, then the U.S. and/or Israel could argue that they have no alternative but to use one of the military options to stop the fundamentalist regime from acquiring the capabilities and fissile materials to develop nuclear weapons.

The Iranian state, under both monarchy and the fundamentalist regime, is a "rentier state," which means that it is highly dependent on oil. As long as the oil income flows into the coffers of the state, the ruling regime enjoys a great deal of autonomy from domestic social classes and domestic pressures. However, if the oil income is stopped, the regime could face serious difficulties in remaining in power.[50] One of the main reasons that the Shah was forced to leave power was the successful strike by workers in the oil fields and refineries. Because repression is far more severe under the fundamentalist regime, where several thousands have been executed in a matter of weeks (e.g., June–December 1981 and September 1988), a level of repression that simply was not in existence under the monarchy, oil workers could not be asked by the opposition to go on strike under a regime that would not hesitate to execute thousands of them to break the strike. Because the oil income cannot be stopped at the point of production, it is, therefore, necessary to stop it at the point of exchange.

According to the Islamic Republic's Central Bank, oil accounts for about 80 percent of foreign earnings, about 60 percent of government revenues, and about 30 percent of GDP.[51] The government received $55 billion in export of oil and natural gas in the 2005–06 fiscal year, in comparison to $23 billion in the 2002–03 fiscal year.[52] With the huge rise in the price of oil, the Iranian government is expected to receive around $100 billion in 2008. All this income goes directly into the hands of the regime. This income allows the fundamentalists to pay for their coercive apparatuses, provide subsidies to maintain the allegiance of their social base, co-opt nonfundamentalists through financial largesse, and prevent the economy from collapse. By purchasing oil and natural gas from the Iranian government, the outside world is helping the fundamentalist regime remain in power. In other words, by purchasing oil and natural gas from the regime, the outside world is having a determining impact on the internal struggles in Iran to the benefit of the fundamentalists and to the detriment of the opposition. Economic sanctions would deprive the fundamentalists of billions of dollars and thus weaken them substantially. This would in effect enable and empower the Iranian people themselves to undermine the fundamentalist regime. The riots in 2007 after the price of gasoline was raised from about 40 U.S. cents a gallon to 50 U.S. cents is an indication of the popular discontent with the economic situation. They also show that the poor do not support the regime and that the regime's hold on the populace is fragile.

Russia and China have opposed tough sanctions against the fundamentalist regime. China's opposition perhaps is based on its need for oil. Oil-hungry China has established significant energy ties with Iran. China is not happy with tension between Iran and the international community, which is a major cause for the dramatic rise in oil prices in the past several years.[53] China would like to see Iran show transparency in its nuclear program and resolve the matter peacefully. China receives more than 14 percent of its imported oil from Iran, and is a major exporter of military hardware and consumer goods to Iran.[54] Some have charged that China deliberately stalls UN Security Council action against the Iranian regime due to its economic relations with Iran.[55]

Oil-exporting Russia has actually benefitted financially from the dramatic rise in oil prices. Russia has had lucrative military contracts with Iran as well as contracts for the reconstruction of the Bushehr nuclear power plant. In addition, Russia benefits from the exclusion of American companies, goods, and services due to American sanctions. Russia benefits from continuing tension between Iran and the United States as long as there are no actual military operations or serious sanctions that would harm its financial trades with Iran. Russia opposes both uranium enrichment by Iran and regime change. After Russia delivered nuclear fuel for the Bushehr nuclear power plant, its foreign minister Sergei Lavrov told the Moscow daily *Vremya Novostei*: "We believe that Iran has no economic need to proceed with its programme of uranium enrichment... We are trying to persuade the Iranians that freezing the programme is to their advantage as it would immediately lead to talks with all countries of the 'six,' including the United States."[56]

The EU is more complicated. In October 2007, the EU foreign ministers failed to agree with new sanctions proposed by French Foreign Minister Bernard Kouchner. The Gordon Brown government has not been as vocal as the Blair government, but seems to be quietly pursuing American policies. In late 2007, the British government explicitly supported tougher UN Security Council sanctions as well as EU sanctions.[57] President Sarkozy has reversed Jacques Chirac's policies and strongly supported both UN and EU sanctions against the Iranian regime.[58] Although initially German chancellor Angela Merkel's government grew closer to the U.S. position and strongly supported the UN Security Council sanctions resolutions, in late 2007 it slightly moved away from the U.S.–U.K.–French position. The center-right government of Silvio Berlusconi has been closer to the U.S. position than the center-left Romano Prodi government that it replaced in May 2008.

Germany and Italy, which have significant trade with Iran, seem to be less willing to go along with stronger sanctions. Italy ranks first among EU countries in total amount of trade (imports and exports), and Germany ranks second. Italy's total trade with Iran reached its height in 2004 with a total of 4,322 billion euro, with much of Iranian exports being oil and gas, and Italian exports being "mechanical machinery and equipment, electric machinery... chemical, metal and metallic products."[59] German annual exports to Iran amount to almost $5 billion.[60]

Russia, China, and many EU countries have lucrative economic relations with Iran. Although the oil needs of several are serious, the actual amount of trade is less than $7 billion for each country. The potential cost of military Options 1–4 would be thousands of deaths and serious disruption to oil supplies, and the potential costs of Options 5, 6, and 7 are the possibility of tens of millions of deaths (in Iran, Israel, and Palestine). By subsuming the comparatively minor economic benefits, the great powers (EU countries, Russia, China) would be serving both their own long-term interests and those of the international community, and also saving the lives of tens of millions of people in Iran, Israel, and Palestine.

To gain their support for UN Security Council comprehensive sanctions, President Barack Obama needs to be able to convince skeptical Russian and Chinese leaders that the U.S. goal in Iran is not economic benefit or crass imperialism, but rather confronting a truly horrific situation. The president also needs to be able to convince the global public of the necessity of economic hardships that such sanctions would entail.

Option 9: Reconfigured Containment

This policy option is based on the assumption that Iran is developing a nuclear weapons program, but that its leaders are fully rational and that mutual assured destruction would prevent them from detonating their nuclear bombs on enemy territory.[61] However, some of those who argue that the world must learn to live with a nuclear-armed Iran advocate that it would be necessary to organize a new alliance against the threat of fundamentalist-ruled Iran and its attempt to impose its hegemony in the region. The constituting elements of this containment would include Sunni Arab states (especially Saudi Arabia, Jordan, Egypt, and the Persian Gulf Arab states), Israel, and the United States. To create this alliance, it would be necessary to resolve the Palestinian-Israeli conflict or at least seriously move toward such a resolution. Many believe that the Annapolis meeting in November 2007 was convened to serve such a purpose. This option regards the American and Israeli nuclear arsenal as sufficient to deter Iran from using its nuclear weapons, but it would be necessary to develop a more robust conventional force as well as diplomatic alliances to counter Iran's growing military and political influence, which the overthrow of Taliban and Baathi regimes in Afghanistan and Iraq brought about.

This option does not preclude negotiations and detente with Iran while maintaining military options and economic sanctions, as was done during the containment of the former Soviet Union. The same flaws that exist for comprehensive negotiations also exist for containment plus negotiations.

This option does not preclude an eventual conventional war between Iran and the rest of the alliance if Iran attempts to extend its influence in the region. A major problem with this option is that it assumes that the fundamentalist regime would not use nuclear weapons even if it were to lose a conventional war and those forces were to cross Iranian borders. This option may inadvertently lead to a nuclear exchange leading to tens of millions of deaths.

Option 10: Naval Blockade

In early 2008, the option of naval blockade gained prominence.[62] Two concurrent resolutions were introduced in the U.S. Congress that implied demands for a naval blockade. The House resolution (H. CON. RES 362) was introduced on May 22, 2008 and the Senate resolution (S. RES. 580) was introduced on June 2, 2008.[63] The House version

> demands that the President initiate an international effort to immediately and dramatically increase the economic, political, and diplomatic pressure on Iran to verifiably suspend its nuclear enrichment activities by, inter alia, prohibiting the export to Iran of all refined petroleum products; imposing stringent inspection requirements on all persons, vehicles, ships, planes, trains, and cargo entering or departing Iran; and prohibiting the international movement of all Iranian officials not involved in negotiating the suspension of Iran's nuclear program . . .

This option is based on the assumption that Iran has a clandestine nuclear weapons program with the possibility of success within one to few years. The naval blockade could serve several purposes. It could compel Russia and China to agree with tough sanctions. It could send a signal to Iran's leadership that the U.S. is serious and willing to move beyond words. But also on its own right, the blockade could cripple Iran's import of refined petroleum and export of crude oil and natural gas.

This option hopes that such a naval blockade may cause: Iran's leaders to suspend uranium enrichment; an immense economic distress that would preoccupy the regime with domestic problems and render it unable to become aggressive overseas; the regime to lose resources for expansion of its nuclear program; the collapse of the economy and the regime; or the regime to initiate a hot war against the U.S. Navy, which it would lose.

If Iran's development of nuclear bomb is imminent (e.g., less than six months), then this blockade would not work. Iran could wait until it assembles the nuclear device and then challenge the blockade.

If the United States and its allies are unsuccessful in convincing Russia and China to agree with comprehensive UN Security Council-imposed sanctions, then this policy could accomplish its intended goal. If Iran did not retaliate violently, then the naval blockade would have the same results as those discussed in Option 8 (UN Security Council comprehensive sanctions). If Iran retaliated violently, that action would provide justification for one of the military options (options 1–4). Therefore, if the United States decides to implement this option, it should also be prepared for the consequences discussed in the military options. It would not be safe to assume that Iran's retaliation would be limited to confrontation with American forces implementing blockade. Knowing full well its huge conventional naval inferiority, Iran is more likely to respond asymmetrically in the Persian Gulf, Strait of Hormuz, in Iraq, and beyond. Just like retaliation against military attacks, Iran may respond by unleashing its proxies, such as the Lebanese Hezbollah, against Lebanon's government, Israel, or in terrorist campaigns in Europe and inside the United States.

The potential benefits of this option are very high. Depending on what forms of response Iranian leaders decide upon and how prepared American planners are for the various contingencies, the costs could vary from insignificant to extremely high.

Option 11: Covert Operations

Proponents of this option argue that a covert campaign of sabotage and assassinations could delay or stop Iran's nuclear program. One of the proponents of this option is Patrick Clawson, who is the deputy director at the Washington Institute for Near East Policy.[64] This policy is not without precedent. It is widely believed that the Mossad, Israel's secret service, was behind a series of assassinations of scientists in Egypt and Iraq, as well as the sabotage of nuclear and missile-related components and programs in the 1950s, late 1970s, and early 1980s.[65] A report written by former Israeli senior military and intelligence officials in 2005 advocated "a swift covert strike against either the 'enemy leadership elites' or the program's scientists and engineers."[66] American news networks have reported that President Bush had authorized the CIA to carry out nonlethal covert actions to undermine Iran's nuclear program.[67] It is unclear whether the 44-year old Ardeshir Hassanpour, one of Iran's top nuclear scientists who was working on the nuclear program, died by accident or was assassinated by Mossad, as alleged by many sources.[68] Some have speculated that Iran's capture of fifteen British marines and sailors in March 2007 was a response to the "cloak-and-dagger" operations involving U.S. and British clandestine operations.[69]

This option is at best a stopgap measure. It carries huge costs and huge risks with only limited short-term benefits. Moreover, it is arguably illegal under international law. If the agents are arrested, serious negative consequences would follow. One may not discount the possibility that the news leaks about covert operations may, in fact, be part of psychological warfare against the regime and not the actual policy being implemented by the United States, the United Kingdom, and Israel.

Option 12: Regime Change via Nonviolent Struggle

The fundamentalist regime has lost its ideological legitimacy and political hegemony, but not its ability to coerce the population into submission. The failure of the reform movement within the fundamentalist oligarchy to bring meaningful reforms, and the failure of the democratic opposition to mobilize the population before the collapse of the reform movement or after its collapse, has made this option seem like a distant past.[70] If the widespread belief among Iranians is true, that the majority of Iranian people wish to see the fundamentalist regime replaced with a secular democratic republic, then one may not totally discount this option. However, as long as the regime is able to sell oil and natural gas, it is able to maintain its social base and coercive apparatuses; therefore, it is able to successfully suppress opposition.

Perhaps UN Security Council comprehensive economic sanctions, political sanctions (such as those imposed on the apartheid regime in South Africa), or naval blockade may weaken the regime to such an extent that they might reinvigorate the opposition. Trade and political rapprochement with the regime increase its resources and decrease the likelihood of transition to democracy.

There is very little that the U.S. government can do to directly help participants in the pro-democracy movement. Any close cooperation would be used by the regime to taint them as collaborators, and thus subject them to severe repression. However, the United States could increase the Voice of America and Radio Farda television and radio broadcasts to provide news and analysis to the Iranian people. These programs are hugely popular among various sectors of the public. They infuriate the fundamentalists and present the views of other groups, including some dissidents.

Conclusion

Had there not been a perception that Iran has a clandestine nuclear weapons program and the perception that deterrence would not work due to the extremist, martyrdom-seeking, and/or apocalyptic nature of the fundamentalist Shia regime ruling Iran, then the wisest policy could have been to stay out of Iranian affairs and let Iranians themselves sort out their politics. If one is convinced that there is no nuclear weapons program or if the world could convince Iran's fundamentalist rulers to verifiably suspend nuclear enrichment programs, then one should stay out of Iranian politics.

The possibility of nuclear weapons in possession of a Shia fundamentalist regime with expansionist and hegemonic ambitions has brought great alarm to several powers. It appears highly unlikely that Israel and the United States would be willing to live with the fundamentalist regime possessing a nuclear weapons capability. The NIE report pushed the decision timeframe from 2008 to 2009–2010. The new American president will face grave decisions. It has become a cliche to state that there are no good options. However, there are worst-case scenarios that could result in the deaths of tens of millions. One should do all one can so that U.S. Senator Hillary Clinton's scenario to "totally obliterate" Iran in an American retaliation of Iran's use of nuclear bombs would not become an actual scenario.

If the Obama administration is not able to persuade other powers to enact comprehensive economic sanctions by the UN Security Council, then Israeli or American military action would be the most likely scenario. If the analysis in this study is correct, other than a global effort via the UN Security Council to push the fundamentalist regime out of power, war would be the result, with horrendous loss of life. The surgical strike option by the U.S. may appear as an easy solution, but its faulty assumption of no retaliation by Iran's rulers could cause great chaos and much harm. The nature and history of Iran's fundamentalist rulers do not leave much room for optimism about prospects of diplomatic agreements (grand or piecemeal) resulting in peace. If the historical pattern of the fundamentalist regime's repeated deceptions is any lesson, such agreements could result in tens of millions of deaths. Potential costs of covert operations are immense and the likelihood of success virtually nil. The noblest policy option, regime change via nonviolent struggle, may not be achieved without the UN Security Council comprehensive sanctions. This would leave naval blockade as the only remaining option if President Obama could not convince Russia and China for support at the Security Council. The naval blockade may either result in regime change by the Iranian people themselves or result in one of the military options.

If the analysis in this study is correct, the decisions to be made on how to deal with Iran by President Obama—as well as those by the leaders of Israel, Russia, China, and the EU—will have a truly major political and historical impact. The wrong decision could result in unprecedented human catastrophe. The right decision could result in harsh criticisms and condemnations from many quarters for many decades. The findings and conclusions of this study may help us further discuss and elaborate various policies. Such elaborations could help increase the likelihood of avoiding the worst-case scenarios and help increase the likelihood of making the best policies possible.

Notes

1. United States, Office of the Director of National Intelligence, National Intelligence Estimate, *Iran: Nuclear Intentions and Capabilities* (November 2007), available at http://www.dni.gov/press_releases/20071203_release.pdf, accessed December 3, 2007.
2. Peter Baker, "Bush's War Rhetoric Reveals the Anxiety that Iran Commands," *Washington Post*, October 19, 2007, A05.
3. Sheryl Gay Stolberg, "Nuclear-Armed Iran Risks World War, Bush Says," *The New York Times*, October 18, 2007.
4. "Cheney: U.S. Will Not Let Iran Go Nuclear," Associated Press, November 20, 2007, available at www.usatoday.com/news/washington/2007-10-21-cheney-iran_n. htm?loc=interstitialskip, accessed November 20, 2007.
5. Ibid.
6. Ibid.
7. "Fact Sheet: Designation of Iranian Entities and Individuals for Proliferation Activities and Support for Terrorism," October 25, 2007, available at http://www.treasury.gov/press/releases/hp644.htm, accessed October 26, 2007. For an assessment of the Bush administration's economic activities towards the Iranian regime, see Ilan Berman, "Toward an Economic Strategy against Iran," *Comparative Strategy*, vol. 27 (January/February 2008): 20–26.
8. Scott D. Sagan, "How to Keep the Bomb From Iran," *Foreign Affairs*, vol. 85 (September/October 2006): 45–59.
9. Joel Greenberg, "Experts: Strike against Iran a Last Resort for Israel," *Chicago Tribune*, December 26, 2007.
10. Efraim Inbar, "The Need to Block a Nuclear Iran," *Middle East Review of International Affairs*, vol. 10 (March 2006): 85-104. According to the BBC, Israel says "repeated statements by

Iran's president that the Jewish state should cease to exist are evidence of an intension to use nuclear weapons against it in the future." "Olmert says Iran still dangerous," BBC, December 11, 2007, available at http://news.bbc.co.uk/2/hi/middle_east/7139526.stm, accessed December 12, 2007.

11. Herb Keinon, "Analysis: The Military Option is Now on the Table," *The Jerusalem Post*, October 19, 2007.

12. Yaakov Katz and Herb Keinon, "Gantz: 'World Doesn't Appreciate Gravity of Iranian Nuke Threat,'" *The Jerusalem Post*, December 17, 2007; Peter Spiegel, "Mullen Reassures Israel on Iran," *Los Angeles Times*, December 11, 2007.

13. Whitney Raas and Auston Long, "Osirak Redux? Assessing Israeli Capabilities to Destroy Iranian Nuclear Facilities," *International Security*, vol. 31 (Spring 2007): 7–33.

14. Ibid.: 13.

15. Michael R. Gordon and Eric Schmitt, "U.S. Says Israeli Exercise Seemed Directed at Iran," *The New York Times*, June 20, 2008.

16. Jamey Keaten, "Europeans Ponder Sanctions against Iran," Associated Press, October 27 2007.

17. Ibid.

18. Kiomars Roshan, "*Qabeliyat Hamele Nezami America be Iran: Az Teori ta Vaqeiyat*" [American Capability to Make Military Strikes on Iran: From Theory to Reality], Radio Farda, November 22, 2007, available at: www.radiofarda.com/Article/2007/11/22/f4_Attack-Iran-US-capability-military.html, accessed November 22, 2007.

19. Keith B. Payne, *Deterrence in the Second Nuclear Age* (Lexington: University Press of Kentucky, 1996); Scott Sagan, "How to Keep the Bomb from Iran," *Foreign Affairs*, vol. 85 (Sept/Oct 2006): 45–59; Bradley A. Thayer, "Thinking about Nuclear Deterrence Theory: Why Evolutionary Psychology Undermines Its Rational Actor Assumptions," *Comparative Strategy*, vol. 26 (July/September 2007): 311–323; and Mehdi Khalaji, *Apocalyptic Politics: On the Rationality of Iranian Policy* (Washington, DC: The Washington Institute for Near East Policy, January 2008), available at http://washingtoninstitute.org/download.php?file=PolicyFocus79.pdf.

20. Norman Podhoretz, "The Case for Bombing Iran: I Hope and Pray that President Bush Will Do It," *Wall Street Journal*, May 30, 2007, available at www.opinionjournal.com/federation/feature/?id=110010139, accessed June 1, 2007.

21. Joshua Muravchik, "Iranian Bomb 'Intolerable,'" *USA Today* online edition, November 20, 2007, available at http://blogs.usatoday.com/oped/2007/11/opposing-view-i.html, accessed November 20, 2007.

22. In the words of Deputy Head of the IRGC's Navy, Brigadier Gen. Ali Fahdavi: "The area of Persian Gulf and strategic Strait of Hormuz is such that a small operation can have a big outcome... The Basiji's culture has the advantage of martyrdom-seeking spirit." Reuters, "Iran Militia Could Disrupt Gulf Waterway: Commander," October 29, 2007.

23. Cited in Scott Peterson, "How Iran would Retaliate if it Comes to War," *Christian Science Monitor*, June 20, 2008. Khamenei's words are from 2006. Regime officials have said the same things numerous times.

24. "Iran Warns of 'Limitless' Response to any Military Strike," Agence France Presse, June 22, 2008.

25. According to Commander of IRGC's Artillery and Missiles, Brigadier Gen. Mahmoud Chaharbaghi: "In the first minute of an invasion by the enemy, 11,000 rockets and cannons would be fired at enemy bases... We have identified our targets and with close surveillance of targets, we can respond to the enemy's stupidity immediately." "Iran to Fire '11,000 Rockets in Minute' if Attacked," Agence France-Presse, October 20, 2007.

26. For comments of Iranians to surprised Western reporters in Iran see: Helena Smith, "Generation Ex-communicated: Iran's Hardline Muslim Leadership is Struggling to Crack Down on the Country's Rebellious Youth," *The Guardian*, September 3, 2002; Tim Judah, "Hardliners in Iran Want to Down US Jets," *The Observer*, August 4, 2002; and Dan De Luce, "Hopes and Fears," *The Guardian*, March 21, 2003.

27. S. Rob Sobhani, "The Prospects for Regime Change," in Patrick Clawson and Henry Sokolski, eds., *Checking Iran's Nuclear Ambitions* (Carlisle, PA: Strategic Studies Institute, U.S. Army War College, 2004) pp. 61–79.

28. See www.carnegieendowment.org/publications/index.cfm?fa=view&id=19677&prog=zgp&proj=zme,znpp.

29. Azadeh Moaveni, "Why Iranians Like America Again" *Christian Science Monitor*, June 3, 2008. Moaveni reports observing a woman in a public bus said loudly: "Let the Americans come . . . Let them sort things out for us." Such public words were very common in Iran between late 2001 and early 2004.

30. See Scott Peterson, "How Iran Would Retaliate if it Comes to War," *Christian Science Monitor*, June 20, 2008.

31. U.S. Government, Department of Energy, Energy Information Administration, "Persian Gulf Region," (June 2007) available at www.eia.doe.gov/emeu/cabs/Persian_Gulf/pdf.pdf, accessed March 25, 2008.

32. Ted Galen Carpenter, "Toward a Grand Bargain with Iran," *Mediterranean Quarterly*, vol. 18 (Winter 2007): 15.

33. Steven Mufson, "Strike on Iran Would Roil Oil Markets, Experts Say," *Washington Post*, October 26, 2007. The figures for 2005 were slightly different. See Charles Robertson and Mark Cliffe, *Attacking Iran* (ING Wholesale Banking Report, January 9, 2007), p. 18. According to the British Petroleum and cited in the ING report, Iran's export was 2.391 million barrels per day, and Saudi Arabia's export was 9.144 million barrels per day.

34. Mufson, "Strike on Iran." ING's report provides slightly different data. The U.S. increased its SPR by 150 million barrels in 2003. Considering that U.S. imports are around 13 million barrels per day, the SPR would provide for 75 days if all oil imports were halted. The closure of the Strait of Hormuz would not impact other major oil exporters such as Russia, Norway, Nigeria, Algeria, Mexico, and Kazakhstan. Only Venezuela has indicated that in case of American attack on Iran, it would stop its oil exports to the United States.

35. George Jahn, "Iran's Use of Oil Weapon Cuts Two Ways," Associated Press, December 1, 2007.

36. Michael O'Hanlon, of the Brookings Institution, is a main proponent of this argument. See Radio Free Europe/Radio Liberty, "Washington's Dilemma: To Negotiate with Tehran or Not?" June 18, 2008, available at http://www.rferl.org/featuresarticle/2008/6/78EDB8A8-08D4-4672-A436-477D9A1414EE.html, accessed June 18, 2008.

37. One of the most forceful advocates of this position is Col. Lawrence Wilkerson (Ret.), former chief of staff to Secretary of State Colin Powell. See his interview at http://therealnews.com/t/index.php?option=com_content&task=view&id=31&Itemid=74&jumival=1628&updaterx=2008-06-07+03:30:51, June 7, 2008, accessed June 17, 2008.

38. For the most sophisticated advocate of this option see: Flynt Leverett, *Dealing with Tehran: Assessing U.S. Diplomatic Options toward Iran*, December 4, 2006, available at www.tcf.org/list.asp?type=PB&pubid=595. For a criticism of this option, see Masoud Kazemzadeh, "The Perils and Costs of a Grand Bargain with the Islamic Republic of Iran," *American Foreign Policy Interests*, vol. 29 (October 2007): 301–327.

39. For the details of the event, including translation of Rouhani's words, see Kazemzadeh, "The Perils and Costs": 318, 325–6.

40. "Quotes from Ayatollah Khomeini," compiled by Jalal Matini, translated by Farhad Mafie, available at http://www.iran-heritage.org/interestgroups/government-article2.htm, accessed June 2, 2008. For quotes of Ayatollah Khomeini's speeches saying one thing before the revolution and then doing the opposite after capturing power, see Ali Gharib, *Eastadeh bar Arman: Ravayat Foroupashi Yek Enghelab*, pp. 8-10, available at http://www.box.net/shared/rkc4biugpb, accessed June 2, 2008. This is in Persian.

41. For example, the fundamentalist regime explicitly asked Germany to swap a German tourist who had mistakenly strayed into Iranian waters for the man who assassinated four Iranian dissidents in Berlin. German officials have reportedly complied and released two convicted members of the

assassination team, Kazem Darabi (Ministry of Intelligence agent) and Abbas Rhayel (member of the Lebanese Hezbollah) on December 10, 2007. The agents were tried for the assassination of three leaders of the Democratic Party of Iranian Kurdistan, including its secretary-general Dr. Sadeq Sharafkandi and a member of Marxist democratic socialist organization United Left Council for Democracy and Independence, Mr. Nouri Dehkordi, in Berlin on September 17, 1992. "Diplomatic Wrangling: Iran Wants Germany to Swap Assassin for Jailed Tourist," *Der Spiegel*, January 15, 2007, available at www.spiegel.de/international/0,1518,459731,00.html, accessed January 16 2007; and "Iran: Terrorist Freed in Germany is Welcomed by Tehran," Radio Free Europe/Radio Liberty, Radio Farda, December 12, 2007.

42. Cited in Therese Delpech, *Iran and the Bomb: The Abdication of International Responsibility* (New York: Columbia University Press, 2007), p. vii.

43. Scott Sagan and Kenneth Waltz, "A Nuclear Iran: Promoting Stability or Courting Disaster?" *Journal of International Affairs*, vol. 60 (Spring/Summer 2007): 135–152.

44. Ibid. The video of the debate between Kenneth Waltz and Scott Sagan, February 8, 2007, held at SIPA, Columbia University, is available at: www.dkv.columbia.edu/demo/video/sipa-nuclear_iran.html, accessed August 1, 2007.

45. For one of the most sophisticated arguments in this genre see Jim Walsh, "Iran and the Nuclear Issue: Negotiated Settlement or Escalation?" Testimony before the Subcommittee on Federal Financial Management, Government Information & International Security Committee on Homeland Security & Government Affairs, United States Senate, July 20, 2006, available at http://web.mit.edu/SSP/people/walsh/Walsh%20test%207-20-06f.pdf, accessed December 21, 2007.

46. This scenario was discussed by Sen. Hillary Clinton when she stated that if Iran were to use nuclear bombs on Israel, the U.S. would "totally obliterate" Iran. Available at http://abcnews.go.com/WN/Vote2008/Story?id=4698059&page=1 (April 25, 2008), accessed April 27, 2008.

47. Masoud Kazemzadeh, "Ahmadinejad's Foreign Policy," *Comparative Studies of South Asia, Africa and the Middle East*, vol. 27 (2007): 423–449; Kamran Scot Aghaie, *The Martyrs of Karbala: Shi'i Symbols and Rituals in Modern Iran* (Seattle: University of Washington Press, 2004).

48. www.oefre.unibe.ch/law/icl/ir00000_.html.

49. Bruce W. Nelan, "Diplomacy of Terror," *Times Magazine Europe* online edition, May 31, 1993, available at www.time.com/time/europe/timetrails/iran/ir930531.html, accessed June 2, 2002; and Thomas Sancton, "Iran's State of Terror," in *Times Magazine Europe* online edition, November 11, 1996, available at www.time.com/time/europe/timetrails/iran/ir961111.html, accessed June 2, 2002.

50. Masoud Kazemzadeh, "The State, Civil Society and the Prospects of Islamic Fundamentalism," *Comparative Studies of South Asia, Africa and the Middle East*, vol. 16 (Fall 1996): 55–67.

51. Economic Research and Policy Department, Central Bank of the Islamic Republic of Iran, "Annual Review 1383," (2004/2005), September 2005, available at www.cbi.ir/default_en.aspx, cited in Elliot Hen-Tov, "Understanding Iran's New Authoritarianism," *The Washington Quarterly*, vol. 30 (Winter 2006–2007), 172, 178.

52. Bill Samii, "Iran: Weak Economy Challenges Populist President," Eurasianet.org, July 23, 2006, available at www.eurasianet.org/departments/business/articles/pp072306.shtml, accessed July 24, 2006.

53. AFX News, "Gates Calls on China to Back Tougher Economic Sanctions Against Iran," November 5, 2007, available at www.forbes.com/markets/feeds/afx/2007/11/05/afx4298700.html, accessed November 6, 2007.

54. Robin Wright, "Deepening China–Iran Ties Weaken Bid to Isolate Iran," *Washington Post*, November 18, 2007.

55. Ibid.

56. Ron Popeski, "Russia Says Iran Needs No Uranium Enrichment," Reuters, December 26, 2007. By "countries of the 'six,'" Lavrov is referring to the five permanent members of the UN Security Council (U.S., Russia, U.K., China, and France), plus Germany, which is usually called "5+1."

57. Kim Murphy, "Europe Faces Tough Choices on Iran," *Los Angeles Times*, October 27, 2007.

58. Ibid.

59. Elisabetta Cavanna, "Handbook for Business Hunters," *Heartland: Eurasian Review of Geopolitics*, vol. 4 (2005), 43–44.

60. "The German Question over Iran," *Christian Science Monitor*, November 21, 2007.

61. For the most sophisticated version see Colin Dueck and Ray Takeyh, "Iran's Nuclear Challenge," *Political Science Quarterly*, vol. 122 (Summer 2007): 189–205.

62. Chuck Freilich, "Too Late To Dissuade Iran?" Middle East Strategy at Harvard blog, April 22, 2008, available at http://blogs.law.harvard.edu/mesh/2008/04/not_too_late_to_dissuade_iran/, accessed June 2, 2008; Yossi Melman, "MAD in the Middle East," *Haaretz*, February 15, 2008, available at www.haaretz.co.il/hasen/spages/954411.html, accessed June 17, 2008; "Punxsutawney Condi," *The Wall Street Journal*, May 28, 2008, A16.

63. For the House version see http://thomas.loc.gov/home/gpoxmlc110/hc362_ih.xml; for the Senate version see http://thomas.loc.gov/cgi-bin/query/z?c110:S.RES.580:

64. Jamie Glazov, "Symposium: The Showdown [with Iran]," FrontPageMagazine, July 29, 2005, available at http://www.danielpipes.org/article/2814, accessed November 2, 2007.

65. Terrence Henry, "The Covert Option," *Atlantic Monthly*, vol. 296 (December 2005): 54.

66. Ibid.

67. Sheila MacVicar, Ashley Velie, and Amy Guttman, "U.S. Working to Sabotage Iran Nuke Program," CBS News, May 23, 2007, available at http://www.cbsnews.com/stories/2007/05/23/eveningnews/main2843582.shtml, accessed May 24, 2007; Brian Ross and Richard Esposito, "Bush Authorizes New Covert Action Against Iran," May 22, 2007, available at http://blogs.abcnews.com/theblotter/2007/05/bush_authorizes.html, accessed May 23, 2007.

68. U.S. Government, Department of Defense, Defense Threat Reduction Agency, *WMD Insights*, vol. 14 (April 2007): 19–23, available at http://www.wmdinsights.com/PDF/WMDInsights_Apr07Issue.pdf, accessed December 26, 2007.

69. Kamal Nazer Yasin, "Cloak-and-Dagger Occurrences Mark Iran's Relations with United States, Britain," Eurasia Insight, April 9, 2007, available at http://www.eurasianet.org/departments/insight/articles/eav040907_pr.shtml, accessed April 10, 2007.

70. Many Western observers confuse the terms "reformist" and "democratic opposition." The former refers to those within the fundamentalist oligarchy who want to reform the system in order to preserve and prolong the system of clerical rule, *Nezam Velayat Faqih*. The most prominent reformist leader has been former president Mohammad Khatami. The democratic opposition refers to those who want to replace the fundamentalist oligarchy with a democracy. It includes organizations such as the Iran National Front and such figures as Ahmad Batebi and Abbas Amir-Entezam. In the past few years, some groups such as the *Daftar Tahkim Vahdat* (Office for the Consolidation of Unity) and some prominent figures such as Akbar Ganji have left the reformist camp and have joined the democratic opposition.

U.S.–Iran Confrontation: Domestic Asymmetrical Ramifications

The U.S. and the Islamic Republic of Iran (IRI) appear to be headed toward a military confrontation in the near future. The war with the IRI may have a serious terrorist dimension on American soil. The leaders of the IRI are extremist violent Shia fundamentalists, who excel at asymmetrical warfare. Conventional warfare constitutes only a very small aspect of the IRI's confrontation with the U.S. Far more significant will be the IRI's asymmetric policies. As part of their strategy, the IRI will probably use massive terrorist attacks on military, economic, and civilian targets within the territories of all those who form the coalition against it. Therefore, one should be concerned about potential terrorist attacks on various targets in the U.S.

Terrorist attacks and plots on American soil by agents of the IRI have been extremely rare. On July 22, 1980, David Belfield (aka Daoud Salahuddin) assassinated Ali Akbar Tabatabai, a prominent opposition figure in Bethesda, Maryland.[1] The assassin has been living in Iran since. He was rewarded with, among many other things, a 35-minute private meeting with Ayatollah Ruhollah Khomeini, the founder and leader of the Islamic Republic. In July 2009, according to the Glendora, California police, as well as U.S. government documents contained in the WikiLeaks, the Iranian government agents had plans to kill dissidents in Southern California (and London).[2] On October 11, 2011, the U.S. government alleged a plot by certain "elements of the Iranian government" to kill Saudi Arabia's ambassador to the U.S. as well as to bomb the Saudi and the Israeli embassies in Washington.[3]

The IRI and its proxies have carried out attacks on Iranian dissidents on European soil, on American targets outside of the U.S., on Jewish targets around the world, on French citizens on French soil, and on Saudi diplomats around the world.[4]

The Iran Human Rights Documentation Center has documented the assassination of 162 dissidents by the IRI outside of Iran.[5] The Iranian government was involved in the attacks on the U.S. Marine barracks as well as the U.S. and French embassies in Beirut in 1983. On the April 18, 1983 attack on the U.S. embassy, 63 were killed. On the October 23, 1983 attack on the U.S. Marine barracks 241 military personnel were killed. In the attack on the French barracks two minutes later the same day, 58 French paratroopers were killed. The FBI officially blamed the Saudi Hezbollah for the bombing of the Khobar Towers in Saudi Arabia which killed 19 American military personnel on June 25, 1996. The Saudi Hezbollah is closely related to the Iranian government.[6] It is also believed that an Iranian proxy, the Lebanese Hezbollah, carried out the attacks on a Jewish center in Buenos Aires on July 18, 1994, which killed 85 people. Earlier WikiLeaks documents on Iraq and Afghanistan revealed that Iranian government agents and proxies killed many Americans in Iraq and Afghanistan.[7]

The Iranian government has successfully used terrorism in its confrontations with France. When serious differences arose between the IRI and France in 1986, the Iranian government used terrorism in that country.[8] In a series of bombings in France in September 1986, more than 100 were killed or wounded. French investigations of the bombings led to Mr. Wahid Gordji (also spelled Vahid Gorji). Mr. Gorji's occupation was listed as translator in the Iranian embassy in Paris, and he did not have diplomatic immunity. However, according to a report in the *New York Times*, Gorji seemed to have the second senior position in the embassy. The Iranian embassy refused to allow the French to question Gorji. The French encircled the Iranian embassy to prevent his escape. The Iranian government retaliated by placing the French embassy in Tehran under siege and demanded to interrogate the French ambassador for hostile acts. The then-Prime Minister Jacques Chirac resolved the dispute with an agreement, which involved France returning to Iran about $700 million as well as allowing Mr. Gorji to return to Iran. Iran had its proxies in Lebanon release three French hostages, and stopped harassment of the French ambassador in Tehran. The wave of bombings in France abruptly stopped after the deal.

A decision was made by Iran's leaders in 1997 to stop the assassinations abroad. Thus, between 1998 and 2005, no such assassinations occurred. The Iranian government's assassinations abroad seem to have re-started in 2005. On February 14, 2005, a massive car bomb in Beirut killed former Prime Minister Rafik Hariri and 22 other people. The UN Security Council established the Special Tribunal for Lebanon (STL) to investigate the assassination of Rafik Hariri and the other 22 killed on that day. In August 2011 the STL indicted four members of the Hezbollah.[9] The Lebanese Hezbollah was created with the help of the IRI. Lebanese Hezbollah, in its organizational charter as well as in practice, considers the Supreme Leader [*Vali Faqih*] of Iran as the Supreme Leader [*Vali Faqih*] of Lebanese Hezbollah.[10]

The Iranian government publicly denies that the arrested assassins have been working for it, despite solid evidence to the contrary. However, the Iranian government has engaged in swaps of these convicted assassins with Westerners held hostage in Lebanon or imprisoned in Iran.[11]

Resurgent Extremism

Ayatollah Ruhollah Khomeini's failure between 1979 and 1989 to overthrow the regimes in Iraq, Saudi Arabia, Lebanon, Egypt, and Bahrain, as well as the terrible cost of the war with Iraq, compelled many in the ruling fundamentalist oligarchy, such as former presidents Ayatollah Ali Akbar Rafsanjani and Hojatolislam Mohammad Khatami, to suspend such aggressive policies, and instead concentrate on rebuilding Iranian economy. The rise of Ahmadinejad in 2005 and the support given him by the Supreme Leader Ali Khamenei between 2005 and mid-2011 resulted in a return to the bellicose policies of Ayatollah Khomeini. The eclipse of Ahmadinejad and the rise of ultra-hard-liners around the Supreme Leader since mid-2011 indicate the emergence of ultra-hawkish and ultra-bellicose elements in Iran's fundamentalist oligarchy as the main decision makers in Iran today.

Americans are shocked by the Iranian President's annual speeches to the UN General Assembly. Ahmadinejad's words do not come as a surprise to those who study the beliefs of the leaders of Iran. The Supreme Leader Ayatollah Ali Khamenei and other powerful figures such as Ayatollah Ahmad Jennati and Ayatollah Mesbah Yazdi hold more extreme views than those expressed by Ahmadinejad. Khamenei is the most powerful member of the oligarchy, while Jennati is probably the second most powerful member. Mesbah is the most erudite member of the oligarchy. Mesbah is one of two or three clerics most likely to become the next Supreme Leader when Khamenei passes away.

Extremely bellicose articulations of the doctrine of hastening the arrival of the 12th Imam have gained currency among some militant fundamentalists since 2005.[12] The most famous fundamentalist strategic analyst in the Islamic Republic is the veteran Islamic Revolutionary Guards Corps (IRGC) officer Hassan Abbasi, who is the Director of the Center for Doctrinal Analysis.[13] Abbasi strongly opposed détente advocated by reformist elements of the ruling oligarchy such as Rafsanjani and Khatami. Abbasi emerged as one of Ahmadinejad's staunchest and most effective defenders between 2005 and mid-2011. Many of Abbasi's terms and policy proposals were adopted by Ahmadinejad. It appears that since the decline of Ahmadinejad since mid-2011, Abbasi has distanced himself from him.

Abbasi explicitly advocates aggressive foreign policy outside of Iran's territory, confrontation with the U.S., and forcing the 12th Imam to appear.[14] Abbasi explicitly states that one could hasten the appearance of the 12th Imam with bellicose foreign policy against the U.S. He calls this doctrine, "*Doctrine Mahdaviyat*" [The Doctrine of Rapture].[15] Abbasi weaves together nuclear weapons, jihad, suicide missions, and hastening the arrival of the 12th Imam.[16] In the past few years a public campaign has been waged to spread stories about Khamenei, having been chosen by the 12th Imam to be the Supreme Leader, that he has personally met with the 12th Imam, and that during his rule the 12th Imam will appear. These testimonies and stories are usually told by clerics.[17] A major part of Abbasi's doctrine is the notion that one should fight outside of one's own homeland. Abbasi has repeatedly supported the use of asymmetrical terrorism against the enemies of the IRI. Abbasi's doctrine of fighting outside of

Iran's border has gained great currency among the ultra-bellicose members of the hard-line faction. Many IRGC commanders have echoed such views in recent times.

It is widely suspected that Iran possesses agents, clandestine cells, and sleeper cells in the U.S. It is also widely suspected that Lebanese Hezbollah possesses cells and sleeper cells in the U.S. To what extent American intelligence and law enforcement agencies have identified all such individuals cannot be known. Americans only know those they have identified; they do not know which cells they have not identified. The Iranian government and Hezbollah suspect that some of their assets have been compromised, but could not be sure which ones have or have not been compromised. These cells and sleeper cells could be used to carry out terrorist activities if a war breaks out (or is about to break out) between the U.S. and Iran.

The IRI's reach has been extremely limited inside the U.S. compared with its massive assets in Europe and the Middle East region. Therefore, it would be safe to assume that the IRI could not sustain a prolonged terrorist campaign inside the U.S. Moreover, due to lack of secure supply lines, the IRI's assets would not be able to possess materials to inflict massive casualties. In the worst-case scenario, in all likelihood the IRI would be able to detonate a few dozen small bombs in malls and other places where civilians gather.

The IRI could maximize the political and psychological effectiveness of its operations inside the U.S. by using their clandestine cells and sleeper cells all at once right before the commencement of the war and/or immediately after the war begins. The objective of the IRI would be to create panic (by inflicting unexpected terrorist explosions) in order to force the American President to cease operations against the IRI and to withdraw American troops from the theater of operations. The U.S. could effectively counter the IRI by a combination of two policies. First, effective measures could be undertaken to discover, disrupt, and dismantle as many clandestine cells and sleeper cells as possible (before and after the war begins). Second, a public awareness campaign could be developed to psychologically prepare the American public for the IRI's possible use of terrorist operations inside the country. The objective of this campaign would be to undermine the psychological shock of the possible terrorist operations. The public could be reassured that such operations would be very limited in duration and destructiveness.

American security, intelligence, and law enforcement agencies possess vast resources and abilities. They are more than a match for the IRI's extremely limited assets in the U.S. With focus and planning, the U.S. could successfully undermine and contain the IRI's terrorist operations in the homeland.

Masoud Kazemzadeh is Associate Professor of political science at Sam Houston State University, Huntsville, USA.

Notes

1. For an excellent extensive description see: no author cited, *No Safe Haven: Iran's Global Assassination Campaign* (New Haven, CT: Iran Human Rights Documentation Center, May 2008), pp. 18–23. The document is available at www.iranhrdc.org/english/publications/reports/3152-no-safe-haven-iran-s-global-assassination-campaign.html?p=1 (accessed December 24, 2011).
2. Drew Griffin and David Fitzpatrick, "CNN Exclusive: Plotter of Foiled 'Hit' Was Allowed to Return to Iran," CNN, February 21, 2011, www.cnn.com/2011/US/02/04/siu.calif.iran.hit.foiled/index.html (accessed October 15, 2011).
3. No author cited, "Two Men Charged in Alleged Plot to Assassinate Saudi Arabian Ambassador to the United States," FBI, October 11, 2011, www.fbi.gov/newyork/press-releases/2011/two-men-charged-in-alleged-plot-to-assassinate-saudi-arabian-ambassador-to-the-united-states (accessed October 11, 2011); and the complaint filed with the Southern District of New York, October 11, 2011, http://s3.documentcloud.org/documents/255899/federal-charges-against-arbabsiar-manssor-and.pdf (accessed October 11, 2011). CNN Wire Staff, "Iranian Plot to Kill Saudi Ambassador Thwarted, U.S. Officials Say," CNN, October 12, 2011, www.cnn.com/2011/10/11/justice/iran-saudi-plot/index.html?hpt=hp_t1 (accessed October 11–12, 2011 on the continuing story).
4. Matthew Levitt, "Iranian Terror Operations on American Soil," Testimony before a joint hearing of the House Homeland Security Subcommittee on Counterterrorism and Intelligence and Subcommittee on Oversight, Investigations, and Management," October 26, 2011, http://homeland.house.gov/sites/homeland.house.gov/files/Testimony%20Levitt.pdf (accessed November 20, 2011).
5. No author cited, *No Safe Haven: Iran's Global Assassination Campaign* (New Haven, CT: Iran Human Rights Documentation Center, May 2008), pp. 18–23. The document is available www.iranhrdc.org/english/publications/reports/3152-no-safe-haven-iran-s-global-assassination-campaign.html?p=1 (accessed December 24, 2011).

6. No author cited, "Khobar Towers Press Release," FBI, Department of Justice, June 21, 2001, www.au.af.mil/au/awc/awcgate/khobar/khobar_fbi.htm (accessed October 14, 2011).
7. Michael R. Gordon, Andrew Lehren, "Leaked Reports Detail Iran's Aid for Iraqi Militias," *The New York Times*, October 22, 2010, www.nytimes.com/2010/10/23/world/middleeast/23iran.html?_r=1 (accessed October 25, 2010).
8. Youssef M. Ibrahim, "France Lets Bombing Suspect Go In Step to Restore Ties With Iran," *The New York Times*, November 30, 1987, www.nytimes.com/1987/11/30/world/france-lets-bombing-suspect-go-in-step-to-restore-ties-with-iran.html (accessed last on December 24, 2011).
9. Special Tribunal for Lebanon, Press Release, "Indictment and its confirmation decision made public," August 17, 2011, www.stl-tsl.org/en/media/press-releases/17-08-2011-indictment-and-its-confirmation-decision-made-public (accessed August 20, 2011).
10. Ahmad Nizar Hamzeh, *In the Path of Hizbullah* (Syracuse: Syracuse University Press, 2004), pp. 30–36.
11. No author cited, *Murder at Mykonos: Anatomy of a Political Assassination* (New Haven, CT: Iran Human Rights Documentation Center, March 2007), www.iranhrdc.org/english/publications/reports/3150-murder-at-mykonos-anatomy-of-a-political-assassination.html (accessed last December 26, 2011). Also see *No Safe Haven: Iran's Global Assassination Campaign* cited earlier.
12. Mehdi Khalaji, *Apocalyptic Politics: On the Rationality of Iranian Politics* (Washington, DC: Washington institute for Middle East Policy, 2008), www.washingtoninstitute.org/pubPDFs/PolicyFocus79Final.pdf (accessed last January 5, 2011).
13. Reza Valizadeh, "Coup-d'Etat? The Iranian Election in Five Acts," PBS, May 27, 2010, www.pbs.org/wgbh/pages/frontline/tehranbureau/2010/05/coup-detat-the-iranian-election-in-five-acts.html (accessed last December 18, 2010).
14. Numerous videos of Abbasi's lectures have been placed on YouTube. For those on the subjects quoted see: www.youtube.com/watch?v=MyVcgHYD8kY and www.youtube.com/watch?v=1LUZQK1g6uo (accessed last January 8, 2011).
15. Abbasi's speech "*Mahdaviyat*" [Armageddon] or [Rapture] or [Apocalypse], June 2008, www.youtube.com/watch?v=GTmsm8AQJQM (accessed June 25, 2008). The speech is placed on YouTube on seven parts. Also see Abbasi's lecture www.irannegah.com/Video.aspx?id=701 (accessed March 20, 2009).
16. For some of these see www.youtube.com/watch?v=weCXdHJj5q4 (accessed March 20, 2009) and www.youtube.com/watch?v=V6_e5OyrqUM (accessed December 1, 2010).
17. Many such testimonies and stories by clerics are contained in the following internet site close to the Supreme Leader, http://salehat.ir/ (last accessed January 9, 2011).

Index

Abrahamic religions 10
Aghazadeh, Gholam Reza 13
agreements 11, 14–15, 24, 42, 44, 81–82, 97–99, 108, 114; nuclear 12, 24, 81–82
Ahmadinejad 6–8, 10, 12, 14–15, 29, 41–42, 63–65, 92, 95, 100–101, 114
al Qaeda 23, 42, 54, 74–78, 80, 82–83, 85
American Foreign Policy 36, 60; interests 60
American grand strategy 74, 78
American officials 28, 82, 102
American policy of referring Iran 64, 99
Aminzadeh, Mohsen 14, 38
Amrollahi, Reza 13
antiappeasement realists 60, 62
appeasement 55, 59, 61–63, 67, 102
Arabs 52–53, 62, 77, 102
armed forces 7–8, 37, 40–41
Ashura, A.D. 31
Assad regime 79–80, 82, 85
asymmetrical warfare 113
Atomic Energy Organization of Iran (AEOI) 13
Azerbaijanis 52–53

Balochis 52–53, 62
Bani-Sadr, Abol-Hassan 2
Battle of Karbala 31
bombings 91, 113–114
Brookes, Peter 60
Bush, George W. 66

Campbell, Kurt 58
centrifuge plans 64, 99
China 8–10, 38, 43, 74, 81–82, 86, 90, 92–93, 100, 102–104, 106, 108
Chirac, Jacques 114
Chollet, Derek 58
Christianity 10
coercive apparatuses 7, 53, 56, 58, 62–63, 93–95, 103, 107
communist groups 52
comprehensive negotiations 11, 27–28, 98, 105
conflicts 2, 6–8, 11, 26–27, 41, 74–75, 78–79, 84, 86, 97–98
constitution 5–7, 36–37, 54–55, 61, 81, 101
containment 11, 59–60, 62, 105; reconfigured 62, 105
conventional warfare 113
Council of Guardians 6, 11, 37, 40
covert operations 106
culture 4, 37, 66, 75

deceptions 28, 64, 98–99
democratic opposition 107
Democratic party of Iranian Kurdistan (DPIK) 53, 56, 84–85
democratic republicans 49–51, 57
democrats, young 50–51
dictatorship, fundamentalist regime 95
diplomatic pitfalls 98
domestic asymmetrical ramifications 113–115

elections 7–9, 11–13, 15, 36–41, 52, 58, 63, 66; presidential 9, 39, 41
estekbar jahani 29
estekhareh (bibliomancy) 25
ethnic minority parties 57
ethnic parties 52–54
EU-3, 14, 24, 42, 64, 99
Europeans 14, 42–43, 64, 66, 99
expediency council 6, 8, 14–15, 41
expedients 2, 8, 13–15, 24, 38–39

factions, expedient 8, 12–13, 38, 44
Fadaian Islam 22–24
fascism 54–55
forces, democratic 57
foreign policy 2–10, 12–15, 20, 26, 29–30, 37, 39, 41, 44, 55, 58–59, 100; adviser 23, 38–39; analysis 3; consequences 44–45; decision making 3–4, 6, 12, 15; statements 20
foreign policy analysis (FPA) theories of 3–5
Friedman, Thomas 66
fuel cycle 43–44
fundamentalist leaders 22, 100
fundamentalist oligarchy 2, 21, 23–24, 38–39, 42, 58, 107

fundamentalist regime 2, 47–50, 52, 54–66, 80–85, 91, 93, 95–97, 100, 102–103, 105, 107–108; capability 61; evil 56; ruling Iran 85, 90
fundamentalist-ruled Iran 105
fundamentalists: former 55; left 8–9, 39; ruling iran 65; students 9, 38, 51
The Future in Islamic Lands 23

gas, natural 56, 98, 103, 106–107
George, Alexander 20
Ghafari, Hojatolislam Hadi 9
Ghalibaf 10, 40–41
grand bargain 47, 49, 55, 58, 62–67, 92, 97–98

hard-liners 2, 7–15, 30, 38, 40, 42, 44, 63, 65; pragmatic 7–8, 10, 12, 14–15, 29
Hojatieh Society 22–23
Hulsman, John 59
human rights 10, 38, 59, 66, 83, 86, 100
Hussein, Saddam 20–21, 47, 76, 79, 102

idealism 4, 30
ideological army 101
ideology, religious 4
Ikenberry, G. John 4
Imam 9, 20, 22–23, 30, 100, 114
income 56, 103
An Indictment against the Western Civilization 23
International Atomic Energy Agency (IAEA) 13–14, 24–25, 42–43, 64, 81–82, 99
international relations 4
international system 3, 29, 74, 78, 83, 86
intra-elite factionalism 8, 38–39
Iran: attack 91, 95; clandestine nuclear weapons program 13, 41; communists 52; constitution and foreign policy 5–6; embassy 113; foreign policy 2–16, 21–23, 25–32, 37–45, 48–67, 75–87, 91–108, 114–116; fundamentalist oligarchy 114; fundamentalist regime in 60, 79–80, 82, 84, 91, 97; fundamentalist rulers 98, 107–108; government 53, 66, 80–81, 84, 94, 97–98, 103, 113–114; government agents 113; grand strategy 2, 77–78; interests in Iraq 48; Kurds 84–85; leaders 91–92, 94, 98, 100–101, 106, 114; leadership 97–98, 106; nuclear program 13–15; Opposition Groups 49, 54–56; people 9, 28–29, 56, 63, 65–66, 83, 94–95, 97, 99, 102–103, 107–108; policies 15; policies, changed 14; politics 41–42, 44, 57, 107; population 84; regime 5, 60, 62, 64, 82, 93, 97, 99, 104; regime invade Bahrain 101; strategy 78; supreme leader Ayatollah 80; violations 86
Iran Human Rights Documentation Center 113
Iranian-armed opposition groups 94
Iranian.com 66
Iranian Kurdistan 53, 84–85, 94–95, 99
Iranian officials 47, 90, 92, 95, 98–99, 102, 105
Iranian Revolution 61, 101
Iranians 3–5, 13, 39, 57–58, 62–63, 65–67, 80, 82, 84, 94–95, 99–100, 104, 107
Iranian territories 48, 101
Iran-Iraq war 77
Iran National Front (INF) 2, 23, 41, 50, 52, 54, 84
Iraq 4, 9–14, 20–21, 30–31, 39–40, 47–48, 52–53, 59, 61–63, 74–80, 82–85, 92–98, 100–102, 105–106, 113–114; and opposed al-Maliki's anti-Sunni chauvinist policies 85; territory 101
Islam 2, 4–5, 10, 22, 25–28, 52, 55, 76–77, 102
Islamic fundamentalism 4, 11, 32, 55
Islamic fundamentalists 30, 32, 42, 55, 59, 61, 76–77; ideologies 4, 55, 75; regime 90
Islamic Iran Participation Front 15, 38–39
Islamic Republic 9, 12, 14, 25–26, 28–29, 39, 44, 47, 49, 113–114
Islamic Republican Party (IRP) 2, 23, 26
Islamic Republic of Iran (IRI) 3, 21, 23, 30, 42, 61, 101, 113–115; perils and costs of grand bargain 47–67
Islamic Republic's Central Bank 56
Islamic Revolutionary Guards Corps (IRGC) 7, 12–13, 15, 37–38, 40–41, 55, 78, 80, 83–85, 91, 93
Islamic State of Iraq and Sham (ISIS) 74, 76–77, 79–80, 82–85
Islamist groups, radical 10
Israel-Palestinian conflict 8
issue-based dialogue 47, 58, 63, 97

Jafaari, Mohammad Ali 12
Jalili, Saeed 7, 12, 39–40
Jennati 12, 14, 114
Joint Comprehensive Program of Action (JCPOA) 11–12, 15, 83
Jomeh, Imaman 41
Jomhuri Irani 39
Jonbeshe Moghavemat Mardomi 54
Jondollah Organization 54
Judaism 10

Karbala 5, 30–32, 100, 102
Karrubi, Mehdi 9
Kashef al Asrar (1943) 23
Keyhan daily 26
Khalkhali, Ayatollah Sadegh 9
Khamanei, Seyyed Javad Husseni 20
Khamenei Ayatollah 4, 20, 82; Foreign Policy Orientation 20–32; leadership 39; and President Mahmoud Ahmadinejad 92; power 12, 40; retreat 12; speech 30
Khamenei, Seyyed Ali Husseni 20
Khatami, Mohammad 2, 6, 9, 38–39, 48
Khoeiniha, Ayatollah Mohammad Moussavi 9

Khomeini, Ayatollah Ruhollah 2, 5, 8–10, 23–26, 37, 39, 41–42, 50, 55, 57, 75, 77–78, 99, 101
Komala 53, 56, 94–95
Koranic verse 61, 101
Kurdish Regional Government (KRG) 76, 84
Kurds 52–53, 62, 76, 84–85, 94
Kurth, James 59–61
Kuwait 47, 76–78, 81–82, 85, 93–94, 101

leadership 2, 8, 37–38, 53, 57, 78
Leverett 47, 58, 63–65
liberal hawks 58, 60, 62
Lieven, Anatol 59

Majles 6–9, 11, 13–14, 37, 40–41, 84
Mashhad 20–22, 53
Masoud, Mohsen 21
Middle East's crises 74–86
military action 10, 80, 90, 92–94, 96–97
military options 90, 92, 97, 100, 102–103, 106, 108
military strikes 11, 62
minister of intelligence 7, 37
Ministry of Foreign Affairs 6
moderate hard-liners 38, 40–41
moderate opposition 85–86
Mohtashami-pour, Hojatolislam Ali Akbar 9
Mojtaba 21, 24
monarchists 22–23, 42, 49, 51, 54–57
monarchy 24, 50, 56–57, 77, 103
Montazeri, Ayatollah Hussein Ali 24
Mostafa 21, 24
Moussavi, Mir Hussein 9, 13, 38–39
Muslim Brotherhood 23, 75–76

National Intelligence Estimate (NIE) report 90–91, 103, 107
national interests 5, 9, 15, 26, 59, 79, 82, 86
National Movement of Iranian Resistance 41, 50
naval blockade 92, 105–108
Nezam Velayat Faghih 6
Nizam Velayat Faqih 2
non-fundamentalists 2, 23
nuclear facilities 58, 62–64, 82, 91–94, 96
nuclear Iran 100
nuclear power plant 14, 104
nuclear program 3, 7–8, 10–15, 25, 28–29, 39, 41–44, 48, 62, 64, 91–94, 97–99, 104–106
nuclear weapons 13, 25, 28, 61, 65, 90–93, 98, 100–103, 105, 107, 114
nuclear weapons program 13, 42, 44, 82, 85, 90, 93, 97–100, 103, 105, 107

Obama, B. 28, 79–81, 85–86; administration 27, 79–83, 86, 90, 103, 108; policies 79–80, 85–86
oil: income 56, 103; purchasing 56, 103
oligarchical nature 5; Iranian regime 5
oligarchy 5–6, 8–9, 14, 21, 23, 26, 29, 36–38, 41–43, 114
Operational Code 20
opposition groups 39, 49, 54–58, 63, 95, 99

Pahlavi, Reza 51, 57, 95
Pakistan 13, 43–44, 86, 94, 97, 101
Palestinian Islamic Jihad (PIJ) 26, 29, 48
people of Iran 26–29
People's Mojahedin Organization of Iran (PMOI) 23, 52, 55–57, 64, 94–95, 99
personality character, Khamenei 24–25
poll 39, 65–66
post-fundamentalist Iran 94
power: actual 5, 7–8, 36–37; constitutional 5–6; evolution of 36–38
powerful members 8, 14, 41, 114
presidency 6–7, 9–10, 13–14, 36–37, 41, 81
president 5–8, 10, 12, 14, 21, 24–26, 28, 36–39, 41–42, 48, 82, 86, 105
presidential elections 2013, 39–41
public opinion 28, 43

Qods Force 40, 78, 91
Qutb 23

radical Islamic fundamentalist revolution 10
Rafsanjani 8, 10, 13–14, 24–26, 30, 36, 39–42, 114
realism 4, 30
reconfigured containment 62, 105
reformist faction 9, 38–39
reformist members 9, 21, 26, 37, 41, 58
reformists 2, 8–10, 12–15, 23–26, 30, 38–40, 58, 65
regime change 28–29, 54, 58, 62, 80, 83, 85, 92–93, 96, 100, 102, 104, 107–108
regime ruling Iran 92; fundamentalist Shia 107
religion 4, 50
revolutionary guards corps, regime elite islamic 53
rivals 9–10, 24
Rouhani, Hassan 2, 7–8, 12–15, 36, 38, 40–45, 64, 99; election 36–45; foreign policy 41–44; policies 44
Russia 25, 38, 43, 74–75, 79, 85, 90–92, 102–104, 108

Saeedi, Hojatolislam Valialmoslemin Ali 12
Safavi, Navab 22–24, 31, 75
Shamkhani, Ali 7
Shariatmadari, Hussein 26
Shia 2, 5, 23, 25, 31, 75–76, 78, 80, 84; extremist regime in Iran 85; fundamentalism 2; fundamentalist leaders of Iran 93; fundamentalist regime 80, 82–83, 107; fundamentalists 31, 75; Kurds 84; regime in Iran 84
Shia-Sunni conflict 2

Shiite regime: Iran 101; in Lebanon and subjugate non-Shiite groups 102
siasat khareji tahajomi 15
Sick, Gary 59
sleeper cells 93, 115
Soleymani 40, 78
Strategic Petroleum Reserves (SPR) 96
strikes 56, 93, 103
Sunnis 2, 5, 23, 52, 62, 75–77, 79–80, 84; fundamentalism 2; Kurds 62, 84
superpowers 77
supreme leader 4, 6–8, 10, 12, 14, 23, 25–26, 36–38, 40–41, 44, 47–48, 55, 58, 92–93, 114; position of 24, 36–37
Supreme National Security Council (SNSC) 6–8, 12–15, 37, 39, 41
surgical strikes 47, 58–59, 90, 92–94
Syria 9, 12, 20, 29, 39, 44, 53, 63, 77–80, 82–83, 85–86

Takeyh, Ray 59
Trump, D.: administration 85; President 83
Turkomen 52–53, 62

United Nations Security Council (UNSC) 10
United States 27–28, 38–39, 43–45, 47–48, 51, 53–54, 56, 58–67, 74–76, 78–80, 83–84, 90–100, 104–107
UN Security Council Comprehensive Sanctions 102
U.S.-Iran Confrontation 90, 113–115

Vatan Emruz 12

war front 21, 24; bloody Iran-Iraq 24
weapons 13, 78, 91, 93, 98, 100, 102

Yemen 11–13, 77–78, 80, 82–83

Zakani 11